UNDERSTANDING SPORTS MASSAGE

SECOND EDITION

Patricia J. Benjamin, PhD

Scott P. Lamp, LMT

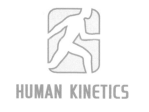

HUMAN KINETICS

Library of Congress Cataloging-in-Publication Data

Benjamin, Patricia J., 1947-
  Understanding sports massage / Patricia J. Benjamin, Scott P. Lamp.--2nd ed.
    p. cm.
  Includes bibliographical references and index.
  ISBN 0-7360-5457-X (soft cover)
  1. Sports massage. 2. Sports physical therapy. I. Lamp, Scott P., 1956- II. Title.
  RM721.B476 2005
  615.8'22'088796--dc22

                                                                    2004019212

ISBN-10: 0-7360-5457-X
ISBN-13: 978-0-7360-5457-7

The Web addresses cited in this text were current as of June 30, 2004, unless otherwise noted.

Acquisitions Editor: Loarn D. Robertson, PhD
Developmental Editor: Jeff King
Assistant Editor: Bethany J. Bentley
Copyeditor: Patsy Fortney
Proofreader: Jim Burns
Indexer: Betty Frizzéll
Graphic Designer: Robert Reuther
Graphic Artist: Tara Welsch
Photo Manager: Kelly J. Huff
Cover Designer: Robert Reuther
Photographer: Kelly J. Huff
Art Manager: Kelly Hendren
Illustrator: Viki Marugg
Printer: Total Printing Systems

Printed in the United States of America.   15   14

The paper in this book is certified under a sustainable forestry program.

Human Kinetics
Web site: www.HumanKinetics.com

United States: Human Kinetics
P.O. Box 5076
Champaign, IL 61825-5076
800-747-4457
e-mail: info@hkusa.com

Canada: Human Kinetics
475 Devonshire Road, Unit 100
Windsor, ON N8Y 2L5
800-465-7301 (in Canada only)
e-mail: info@hkcanada.com

Europe: Human Kinetics
107 Bradford Road
Stanningley
Leeds LS28 6AT, United Kingdom
+44 (0)113 255 5665
e-mail: hk@hkeurope.com

Australia: Human Kinetics
57A Price Avenue
Lower Mitcham, South Australia 5062
08 8372 0999
e-mail: info@hkaustralia.com

New Zealand: Human Kinetics
P.O. Box 80
Mitcham Shopping Centre, South Australia 5062
0800 222 062
e-mail: info@hknewzealand.com

E3206

CONTENTS

LIST OF FIGURES

LIST OF TABLES

LIST OF HISTORY BRIEFS

The use of sports massage has increased dramatically since *Understanding Sports Massage* was first published in 1996. Sports massage has become a valued part of the training routines of Olympic and professional athletes, as well as in school and university sports programs, at health clubs, and among unaffiliated "weekend warriors." It enriches conditioning programs, helps athletes prepare for and recover from competition, reduces the potential for injuries, and aids in injury rehabilitation. Ultimately, sports massage enhances performance.

Although trainers and athletes in the first half of the 20th century commonly used massage, it had virtually disappeared from the sports scene in the United States between 1950 and 1970. An increasing number of sport professionals are now being trained in massage and its applications for athletes.

Athletic trainers and sport physical therapists have found their niche in the prevention, treatment, and rehabilitation of injuries, and many utilize sports massage as an adjunct modality. The integration of these three sport professions provides an optimal health care environment for athletes.

Because sports massage also includes nonmedical applications, coaches and athletes themselves can use simple techniques. Self-massage and partner massage are easy to learn.

The purpose of this book is to show sport professionals how to incorporate sports massage into their athletes' training and health care programs. This book is written for coaches, athletic trainers, sport physical therapists, and sport physicians and chiropractors interested in learning more about sports massage and how it benefits athletes.

Understanding Sports Massage, Second Edition can also serve as a textbook in sports massage training programs. Although hands-on skills are best learned from an experienced sports massage specialist, this book provides the fundamental theory for understanding sports massage today.

The nature of sports massage, its theoretical and scientific underpinnings, and its varied applications are explored in chapter 1, "Theory and Science of Sports Massage." Research citations have been updated in this edition. A section was also added on the implications of massage for athletes taking various medications and drugs. Scientific and experiential evidence is presented in the context of the whole athlete for better understanding of the positive physiological and psychological effects of massage. History briefs reveal a rich tradition of massage for athletes.

On the practical side, individual sports massage techniques are described in detail along with their use and intended effects in chapter 2, "Techniques and Basic Skills." In addition to basic massage techniques, this chapter includes an expanded section on joint movements and stretching, as well as descriptions of the specialized massage techniques of positional release, trigger-point therapy, myofascial massage, and lymphatic-drainage massage. Included are many useful suggestions and ideas on ways that coaches and athletes can use massage for training and performance.

In chapter 3, "Restorative Sports Massage," recovery massage and sample recovery routines without the use of oil are described. This edition features additional remedial and rehabilitative applications of sports massage. Chapter 4, "Sports Massage at Athletic Events," presents guidelines for the use of massage in pre- and postevent situations, including first aid for thermal injuries and muscle cramps. The descriptions in chapter 5, "Maintenance Sports Massage," have been enhanced to show how remedial applications are worked into basic massage sessions for recovery. Remedial applications for the low back, thigh, knee, and neck have been added, as well as an example of a case referred for diagnosis.

Chapter 6, "Planning and Giving Sports Massage," explains the finer points of organizing a session. In addition, it covers body mechanics, palpation, technique selection, and aspects of technique performance such as rhythm and pacing, monitoring pain, and the massage routine. In this edition we renew our commitment to the whole-athlete model as the most effective approach to sport health care and planning sports massage sessions, and we discuss our objections to sport-specific routines. The Trouble Spots Body Chart has been redesigned to be more useful for individualizing sports massage, and the discussion of topical substances used in massage has been expanded. The concept of the optimal therapy zone (OTZ) serves as a useful guide when applying remedial and rehabilitation applications of sports massage.

Chapter 7, "Implementing a Sports Massage Program," explains how sports massage specialists cooperate with other sport and health professionals to provide the best possible care for athletes. The sports massage settings described have been updated to include the integrative sports medicine clinic as well as school programs, health clubs, and private massage practices.

Special features have been added to the second edition of this book to make it more useful to teachers and students. Readers will also be able to locate key information more easily. Features include figures, tables, and lists of history briefs. Each chapter has learning outcomes, and study questions. The design of the book has been upgraded; to show massage techniques more clearly, we've replaced line drawings with photos.

Understanding Sports Massage is written for sport professionals and the athletes they serve. We hope you find it useful for understanding how sports massage can enhance your athletic program.

Patricia J. Benjamin and Scott Lamp
August 2004

ACKNOWLEDGMENTS

The authors would like to thank all those who gave their encouragement and support to this project. Special thanks go to Lee Stang and Mike Fratto for their interest in this revision and willingness to read drafts and offer suggestions. The massage therapists and athletes who posed for the new photographs include Nancy Benjamin, Hoon Kim, Dylan Lott, and Neel Watkins. We appreciate their patience, skill, and professionalism. Logistical support for photography was provided by the Pacific College of Oriental Medicine, Chicago campus. The critical eye of Martha Fourt was welcomed for the final review of the 2nd edition manuscript. Thanks also to those who helped with the first edition, including sports massage therapists Patricia Archer, Jill Bielawski, Robert King, Marge MacLeod, Nikki Nicodemus, and Benny Vaughn for sharing their expertise and suggestions for the book; Victoria Carmona; Alicia Davis, Deb Doricchi, Martha Griffin, Rick Haesche, and Susan Taff from the Connecticut Center for Massage Therapy for their help in preparing initial illustrations. Our gratitude also goes to the countless athletes and sports massage specialists who have kept the tradition of sports massage alive and added to its body of knowledge over the years.

CHAPTER 1

THEORY AND SCIENCE OF SPORTS MASSAGE

LEARNING OUTCOMES

1. List the five major applications of sports massage.
2. Understand the role of the sports massage specialist.
3. Describe the whole-athlete model.
4. Explain how massage enhances athletic performance.
5. Present evidence for the efficacy of sports massage.
6. Identify contraindications and cautions related to sports massage.
7. Be aware of the dangers of doping related to sports massage.

DEFINITION OF SPORTS MASSAGE

Massage refers to the systematic manipulation of the soft tissues of the body for therapeutic purposes. Sports massage is a specific application of massage. Sports massage is the science and art of applying massage and related techniques to maintain the health of the athlete and to enhance athletic performance.

A coach kneading an athlete's shoulders before an event, a trainer frictioning a player's calves during a time-out, a sport physical therapist using deep transverse friction for rehabilitation, and a massage therapist stroking and kneading tired legs at a marathon finish line—these are all examples of sport professionals using massage to address the athlete's unique needs. Similar scenes have occurred in sport arenas since ancient times and attest to the enduring value of massage for athletes.

In this book we explore the applications of massage in various sport settings, describe commonly used techniques, and discuss the theory behind the practice. We present simple massage applications that coaches and athletes can use every day. Athletic trainers and sport physical therapists will learn ways to use massage not only to treat injuries but also to enhance performance. Massage therapists will find a comprehensive survey of the current theory, techniques, and applications of sports massage.

THE MANY USES OF MASSAGE IN SPORTS

Massage is a method that some coaches use to bring out an athlete's best performance. For example, a coach may knead an athlete's shoulders prior to competition for a number of reasons. He may be attempting to warm the muscles, increase circulation, relieve muscular tension, or reduce precompetition anxiety. The coach may also be reassuring the athlete, using touch to elicit a state of calm and to generate greater focus. (See figure 1.1.)

Athletic trainers and sport physical therapists typically use massage for rehabilitation in the tradition of physiotherapy. In this context, massage is one of many modalities for treating injuries. Massage is used in the treatment of conditions such as tendinitis, strains, sprains, and adhesions.

An athlete may use self-massage for general conditioning, to loosen tight muscles, to facilitate stretching, or to prepare for an event. Athletes can also learn to use simple massage techniques on each other.

Following is a list of the five major applications of massage in sports. The first three applications are restorative; their goal is to return an athlete to optimal condition. The last two are related to the athlete's training and competition schedule.

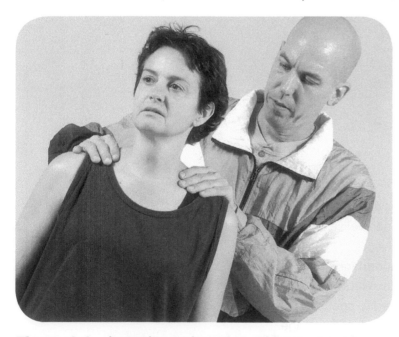

Figure 1.1 A coach may knead an athlete's shoulders prior to competition to help reduce anxiety.

1. Recovery—To enhance the athlete's physical and mental recovery from strenuous sport activity
2. Remedial— To improve a debilitating condition
3. Rehabilitation—To facilitate healing after a disabling injury
4. Maintenance—To enhance recovery from strenuous exertion, to treat debilitating conditions, and to help the athlete maintain optimal health
5. Event—To help the athlete prepare for or recover from a specific competitive event. Event sports massage has three subapplications:

> Pre-event—To help prepare the athlete physically, mentally, and emotionally for an upcoming event
>
> Interevent—To help the athlete recover from an event while preparing for the next round, heat, or trial
>
> Postevent—To help the athlete recover from an event and either to administer first aid or refer problem conditions to another health professional

THE SPORTS MASSAGE SPECIALIST

Massage is the primary focus of sports massage specialists. Their role is to apply massage and related techniques to contribute to the health and safety of athletes and to enhance their performance.

How do sports massage specialists fit into the sport setting? Their role can be compared to that of the coach. Coaches work with the unique talents and physical abilities of each athlete to bring out the best possible performance. Coaches interact with their athletes on a regular basis; they set practice and training regimens, teach and fine-tune technique, give encouragement, and guide athletes through competitions. Although coaches cannot guarantee winning performances, the application of effective coaching methods increases the athlete's performance potential. The actual performance is a complex phenomenon not easy to explain, but it is clearly influenced by the coach.

Sports massage specialists share the coaches' goal—to increase performance potential. They help athletes stay in top physical and psychological condition, prepare for competition, recover from strenuous activity, and keep a positive outlook. Sports massage specialists are most effective when they build ongoing relationships with athletes and become part of the regular support team. (See figure 1.2.)

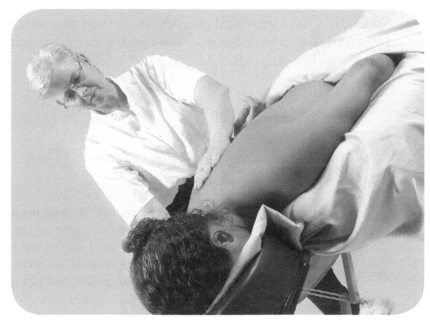

Figure 1.2 Sports massage specialists share the coaches' goal to increase the athlete's performance potential.

Sports Massage Revival c. 1970s

Massage was an essential skill of an athlete's trainer after the revival of the Olympic Games in 1896. But by the 1950s, it had largely disappeared from the U.S. sport scene. Massage for athletes experienced a comeback in the United States in the 1970s after a 20-year hiatus.

Sports massage regained credibility among runners when Lasse Viren, "the Flying Finn," set a world-record time in the 10K and an Olympic record in the 5K at the 1972 Summer Olympic Games in Munich. Runners learned that Viren received deep massage daily—a discovery that sparked interest in sports massage among U.S. athletes. Its use by other high-profile athletes called attention to the once forgotten training aid.

The publicity around Viren and massage came at a time when a growing number of amateur athletes were running 10K events, marathons, and triathlons. Many sought sports massage from massage therapists, a profession going through its own renaissance at the time.

The American Massage Therapy Association (AMTA) set standards for sports massage and established the AMTA Sports Massage Team, which made its first appearance at the Boston Marathon in 1985. Since then, teams made up of specially-trained massage specialists have provided pre- and postevent massage for athletes at local, national, and international events. Sports massage has been available at the Olympics since the 1984 Games in Los Angeles.

THE WHOLE-ATHLETE MODEL

The whole-athlete model acknowledges that athletes bring the totality of their lives to their sport participation. To fully understand the value of massage in enhancing sport performance, we must give up the old metaphor of the athlete as a machine (the mechanist model) and accept the broader view of the whole athlete.

In the whole-athlete model, the sport participant is viewed as a complex physical, mental, emotional, and social being. Athletes must meet the demands of the sport as well as interact with the external environment. The quality of an athletic performance is determined by the synergistic interaction of the parts of the whole system—both the internal and external factors. (See figure 1.3.)

Central to the whole-athlete concept is the idea that a change in any part of the system affects the person as a whole. For example, on a purely physical level, all tissues and systems of the body are connected so that they are affected by the health and activity of all other tissues and systems. This is especially true for systems that pervade the body such as the integumentary, nervous, circulatory, lymphatic, and musculoskeletal systems, and the myofascial tissue that connects them all.

In addition, changes in physical condition affect the mental and emotional state, and vice versa. An example in sport is when muscular aches and pains disturb an athlete's concentration, or when anxiety causes muscle tension that interferes with fluid or graceful movement.

The athlete's relationships with other athletes, coaches, team physicians, athletic trainers, sports massage specialists, staff, and other members of the support team are important components of the whole system. These relationships can have a profound effect on the mental, emotional, and physical state of the athlete. They can affect the group dynamics of the sport setting and ultimately influence individual performances.

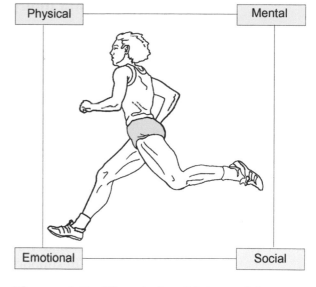

Figure 1.3 The whole-athlete model.

External factors in the sport environment such as training and competition schedules, traveling, facilities, and equipment are also important considerations. To complete the picture, we must add family and friends; school and work; and even community, national, and global situations. In summary, athletes and their performances are affected by a multitude of internal and external interconnected factors.

SPORTS MASSAGE AND ATHLETIC PERFORMANCE

Massage is used for a variety of reasons by different sport professionals. Because massage works on so many levels (i.e., physical, mental, emotional, social), it is a useful approach in addressing the whole athlete.

Exactly how does sports massage enhance athletic performance? It is not a magic bullet that instantly shaves seconds off a 400-meter run, or improves a player's scoring record. Rather, sports massage applied skillfully increases performance potential in three major ways:

1. It optimizes positive performance factors while minimizing negative ones.
2. It decreases injury potential.
3. It supports soft tissue healing.

Optimizing Performance Factors

Sports massage optimizes positive performance factors such as healthy muscle and connective tissues; normal range of motion; high energy; fluid and pain-free movement; and mental calm, alertness, and concentration. It helps minimize negative performance factors such as dysfunctional muscle and connective tissue, restricted range of motion, low energy, staleness, pain, and anxiety.

Positive performance factors are enhanced over a period of time with regular maintenance sports massage. Pre-event and interevent massage contribute to physiological and psychological readiness and provide a last-minute tune-up just before performance.

Decreasing Injury Potential

Sports massage decreases the potential for injury. It is most effective in helping to prevent acute injuries resulting from abnormal tissue conditions (e.g., muscle tears in tight muscles) and chronic injuries caused by repetitive strain (e.g., tendinitis).

One of the most basic benefits of regular sports massage comes from the routine and direct palpation of tissues. Massage practitioners can monitor subtle changes in the condition of tissues and locate potential trouble spots during massage before athletes become consciously aware of them. Especially in the case of chronic injury, an athlete will feel pain with the pressure applied during massage before the injury has progressed to the point of pain in the absence of pressure. Thus, massage can uncover injuries at the subclinical level that can be addressed before they progress to the clinical stage.

When an injury does occur, sports massage specialists join the entire health care team in supporting the athlete's rehabilitation and recovery. The goal is to help the injury heal as quickly and effectively as possible and to minimize side effects and the possibility of reinjury.

Supporting Soft Tissue Healing

Massage contributes to soft tissue healing in a number of ways. For example, circulatory massage brings healing nutrients to the injury site and removes cellular debris. Lymphatic drainage massage reduces primary edema and the possibility of secondary injury caused by pressure from increased fluid in the area

---

HISTORY BRIEF 2

H. Joseph Fay c. 1916

H. Joseph Fay, an Australian authority on massage for athletes, wrote *Scientific Massage for Athletes* in 1916. After commenting on the successes of the American and Swedish athletes who received regular massage, he lamented the poor attitude toward massage in England. Fay described massage for athletes in England at the time as light rubbing, ticklish, and lacking a system.

What is massage as those countries know it who have been successful in international contests? It is the systematic treatment of muscle not lightly but vigorously to bring about definite results. These are: 1. To rid the muscle of waste or poisonous substances which are collected in its depths, and which bring about fatigue and stiffness. 2. To produce additional growth of muscle and bone . . . . (pp.17-18)

The difference between an average trainer and a practical one is that the former merely pats or plays with the hide, while the latter works the meat, or muscle, between the hide and the bone so that it is in its highest state for exercise. (p. 20)

of trauma. Relaxation massage promotes healthy immune system functioning. Deep friction massage promotes the formation of healthy scar tissue and prevents and breaks connective tissue adhesions at the injury site.

Sports massage enhances athletic performance through the effects of massage and related techniques, both at the time of application and accumulated over a period of time. Understanding the science of sports massage is the subject of the remainder of this chapter.

EVIDENCE FOR EFFECTIVENESS

Testimonials about the benefits of sports massage from enthusiastic athletes and anecdotal evidence to support its use for training and competition are abundant. But explaining how massage enhances athletic performance in scientific terms is a challenge. Although the question seems simple, the answer is as complex as the athletes who engage in sports.

What does research tell us about sports massage? Research dealing directly with sports massage is limited. However, studies on the effects of massage in other contexts can shed light on the topic. These studies taken together, and from the perspective of the whole athlete, offer some understanding of how sports massage influences athletic performance.

Limitations of Current Research

Unfortunately, much of the research on sports massage has been done from a mechanistic perspective with a focus on pre-event applications—looking for the magic bullet to improve performance. Predictably, this type of research finds little evidence that a massage given before an event improves the performance immediately following (Boone, Cooper, & Thompson, 1991; Harmer, 1991). These studies are too narrow in scope to explain the more complex phenomenon of the whole athlete.

In addition, sports massage research has done little to acknowledge the mind–body connection. In fact, athletes have been cautioned that "the recuperative benefits [of sports massage] may be more psychological than physiological" (Boone, Cooper, & Thompson, 1991, p. 51). From the whole-athlete perspective, the interplay of mind and body cannot be ignored without severely limiting our understanding of human performance. The psychological effects of massage, the subtle effects of touch itself, and the relationship between the person performing the massage and the athlete have also been largely ignored or discounted.

Kresge (1983) offered further explanation of the limitations of experimental research to account for the effectiveness of sports massage:

> It has been frequently noted that clinical results of massage are often more dramatic than experiments with massage would indicate. Massage, however, tends to have a cumulative effect that is not shown in short-term experiments. It is a science and art combining a variety of strokes in infinite ways to best suit individual situations, while scientific experiments must employ standardized, repeatable procedures. (p. 370)

Cumulative effects over time, the uniqueness of each application of sports massage to a specific athlete, and the characteristic synergy of sport performance make it difficult to design and carry out valid experimental research showing a simple cause-and-effect relationship of massage to sport performance.

Contrary to the mechanistic perspective, massage practitioners are admonished by Juhan (1987) to

> resist the tendency to focus our attention upon localized and objectively predictable effects, and must always strive to include ever broadening and more complexly interrelated processes in our ways of thinking and working. . . . Whatever we do with our hands must be done with the knowledge clearly in mind that all of the physical and mental elements within the human being are inextricably related. (p. 90)

With the whole athlete in mind, we will proceed to examine research on the various physiological and psychological effects of massage, and propose a theory of how they combine to enhance athletic performance. Beyond its simple predictable effects, the ultimate influence of massage on actual athletic performance depends on its integration into the total athletic experience.

CONSTELLATION OF EFFECTS

Sports massage techniques produce a constellation of primary and secondary effects that either influence performance immediately or have a cumulative effect over time. These effects are best viewed as complex interrelated phenomena. To begin to understand what is happening in sports massage, we will use the metaphor of a chain reaction. (See figure 1.4.)

In this chain reaction, sports massage produces primary effects (e.g., improved blood circulation) that bring about secondary effects (e.g., better cellular nutrition or faster recovery) that optimize positive performance factors (e.g., by allowing for longer and more intense practice, massage increases performance potential). In another example, greater elasticity of connective tissue leads to greater range of motion and power, thereby enhancing performance; or, the relaxation response may reduce precompetition anxiety leading to better concentration and better performance.

Example:

Improved blood circulation → better cellular nutrition → faster recovery

More elastic connective tissues → greater range of motion → more power

Less anxiety → greater mental focus → better concentration

Figure 1.4 Chain reaction of the effects of sports massage.

These simplified examples show the interrelationship of effects. Several secondary effects may result from one primary effect of massage. For example, an increase in blood circulation (primary effect) can also increase the removal of metabolites, decrease edema, and hasten the repair of microtraumas (secondary effects). Table 1.1 shows examples of important primary and secondary effects of sports massage.

These primary and secondary effects interact in complex ways. The constellation of massage effects occurs in the context of the whole athlete and therefore also interacts with factors such as coaching, training, and the competition schedule. To apply sports massage for the best results, practitioners must understand as much as possible about each primary and secondary effect; their relationships to each other; and their influence on the athlete's health, well-being, and performance. Practitioners must also be skilled in choosing and performing the techniques that will bring about the desired results based on the needs of the individual athlete.

Table 1.1   Important Primary and Secondary Effects of Sports Massage

Primary effects refer to physiological and psychological changes in the athlete as a direct result of massage. Primary effects include the following:
Improved fluid circulation
Muscular relaxation
Separation of muscle and connective tissue
Formation of healthy scar tissue
Connective tissue normalization
Deactivation of trigger points
General relaxation
Anxiety reduction
Increased feelings of well-being
Increased alertness and mental clarity
Secondary effects refer to performance-related outcomes resulting from the primary effects of massage. Secondary effects include the following:
Greater energy
Freer movement at joints
Faster recovery
Pain reduction
Appropriate level of emotional stimulation
More positive outlook and motivation

Primary Effects

The primary effects of massage include its influence on various physiological and psychological functions of the body and mind, and on the condition of specific tissues. Some of the primary effects of particular interest in sports massage include improved blood and lymph circulation, muscular relaxation, separation of muscle and connective tissues, formation of strong mobile scar tissue, connective tissue normalization, deactivation of trigger points, general relaxation, anxiety reduction, feelings of well-being, and increased mental alertness. These effects are called primary because they directly influence the athlete's condition.

It is important to remember that the general term *massage* refers to a variety of techniques that differ widely in their applications and effects. A specific massage technique or combination and sequence of techniques might have one effect, and a different set of techniques could have a totally different effect. The effects of specific massage techniques are described in greater detail in later chapters.

Improved Fluid Circulation

Good circulation is essential to bring nutrients to muscles and other organs for top athletic performance, and to remove the metabolic by-products of intense physical activity. Improved blood and lymph circulation are well-known primary effects of Western massage.

Several mechanisms may be involved in the application of massage to increase circulation. Increased blood circulation may result from the direct mechanical effects on the vessels and movement of fluids, from the release of vasodilator chemicals, or from "circulatory changes elicited by reflex responses of the autonomic nervous system to tissue stimulation" (Yates, 2004, p. 39).

Massage techniques applied specifically to increase fluid circulation include superficial friction, sliding strokes, kneading, and rhythmic compression. These techniques are applied in combination for best results. Sliding strokes on the arms and legs are performed in the direction from distal to proximal.

Research has consistently demonstrated the increase in lymph flow in normal tissues during massage (Yates, 2004). Specialized techniques of lymphatic drainage massage are designed to maximize the circulation of lymph fluid into lymphatic capillaries, and in the direction of normal lymph flow (Benjamin & Tappan, 2005).

Muscular Relaxation

The repetitive contraction of muscles during physical activity, and the intensity of all-out effort during competition often result in tight and tense muscles. Muscular relaxation occurs during massage when a hypertonic or tense muscle returns to normal tone or to a temporarily flaccid state.

Muscular relaxation may be induced through several different mechanisms. For example, it occurs as part of the general relaxation response of the parasympathetic nervous system as described later. It may also result from a conscious letting go of muscle tension as an athlete assumes a passive role in allowing the practitioner to freely manipulate soft tissues and joints.

Yates (2004) postulated that muscle relaxation may also be due in part to the increased sensory stimulation that happens during massage.

Massage causes a massive increase in sensory input to the spinal cord, so widespread readjustments in these integrated reflex pathways can be expected. It seems reasonable that such a perturbation would spontaneously result in renormalization of imbalances of tonic activity between individual muscles and muscle groups. Thus, where elevated tone has developed in a specific muscle relative to other muscles, because of influences like a sustained posture or emotional state, and has persisted beyond its original cause, the effectiveness of massage may be due in part to increased sensory stimulation. (p. 51)

Juhan's (1987) concept of functional unity of the musculature is also important to keep in mind. Muscles are commonly described as separate anatomical units, but their functioning is best understood as an intricate interplay of muscular tension and release, with synergistic and antagonistic relationships among muscle groups.

That is to say that if I pull on any part of a woven fabric, I create a pull over the entire warp and woof. . . . We almost never find a single discrete muscle that is tense. Rather, we will find areas of tension, or body-wide patterns of tension, whose boundaries do not necessarily follow the anatomical divisions of muscle compartments. And we will never release [relax] a single muscle, but rather we will increase a range of motion that involves several, or many, separate compartments. (p. 113)

Massage techniques used specifically to elicit muscular relaxation include sliding and kneading applied rhythmically and in combination to increase circulation and sensory input. Free joint movements such as rocking and jostling also contribute to sensory input as well as encourage conscious relaxation. Contract–relax stretching results in specific muscle relaxation and elongation. Manual techniques used to address muscle cramps include direct compression, mild stretch, approximation, and reciprocal inhibition.

Separation of Muscle and Connective Tissue

The graceful motion of athletic performance is facilitated by muscle and connective tissues that slide over each other as movements are executed. Any "sticking" of tissues to each other will interfere with smooth motion and limit range of movement. Certain massage techniques are designed to prevent adhering tissues and to break adhesions that develop.

The separation of muscle and connective tissue is achieved through the mechanical actions of lifting and broadening, as well as by applying a focused shearing force across the parallel organization of muscle and tendon fibers. The shearing action breaks connections, or adhesions, made between muscle and connective tissues such as fascia, tendons, and ligaments. It "unsticks" any adhering that would inhibit smooth and flowing movement.

Techniques that separate adhering tissues include skin rolling, kneading, deep transverse friction, and broadening techniques. Specialized myofascial techniques are specifically designed to release restrictions caused by adhering fascial tissues.

Formation of Healthy Scar Tissue

Athletes experience both minor and major soft tissue injuries in the course of training and competition. Proper healing of tissues including healthy scar formation is essential for returning injured athletes to optimal condition. Massage can play an important part in this process.

During the remodeling, or scar maturation, phase of soft tissue healing, massage can provide the soft tissue mobilization needed to create strong yet supple scar tissue. During scar formation, collagen fibers are first arranged randomly to form a weave or path to repair tissue damage. At a later stage, the scar begins to rearrange itself along the direction of stress or line of pull of the muscle.

The mechanical action of deep transverse friction helps produce scars with more parallel fiber arrangement and fewer transverse connections that limit movement. James Cyriax, a well-known champion of deep friction, reasoned that the best way to break interfibrillary adhesions is by forcibly broadening the tissues, which is best accomplished through deep transverse friction. This technique is effective for muscle fibers, tendons, and ligaments (Cyriax & Cyriax, 1993).

Connective Tissue Normalization

The condition of connective tissue can have a profound effect on the ability of the body to move with speed, power, and grace. Connective tissue is found in the fascia that surrounds individual muscles and muscle fibers, and forms ligaments and tendons. It possesses a property called thixotropy by which it becomes "more fluid when it is stirred up and more solid when it sits without being disturbed" (Juhan, 1987, p. 68).

Under chronic stress or chronic immobility, connective tissue tends to become rigid and to lose its flexibility and stretchability. Because of its interconnectedness with surrounding and even remote tissues, connective tissue in poor condition can inhibit overall movement. The chronic stress of intense training can negatively affect connective tissue. The mechanical action of massage is ideal to remedy this situation.

> By means of pressure and stretching, and the friction they generate, the temperature and therefore the energy level of the tissue has been raised slightly. This added energy in turn promotes a more fluid ground substance which is more sol and ductile, and in which nutrients and cellular wastes can conduct their exchanges more efficiently. . . . Skillful manipulation simply raises energy levels and creates a greater degree of sol (fluidity) in organic systems that are already there but behaving sluggishly. (Juhan, 1987, pp. 69-70)

The formation of abnormal collagenous connective tissue, called fibrosis, is curtailed with massage techniques such as kneading, deep friction, and stretching. Healthy connective tissue is the result of maintaining a more fluid ground substance combined with the prevention and breaking of adhesions.

Trigger Point Deactivation

Repetitive strain, poor posture and body mechanics, and trauma are common problems for athletes, which can lead to trigger points (TrPs) in muscles and tendons. In addition to pain, TrPs are accompanied by restricted range of motion, weakening of the maximum contractile force of the affected muscles, and muscle tension in the immediate area—all factors that inhibit optimal performance.

Myofascial trigger points (TrPs) are felt as taut bands of tissue in muscles and tendons, and are tender when pressed. Travell and Simons (1983) defined trigger points as follows:

. . . a focus of irritability in a tissue that, when compressed, is locally tender and, if sufficiently hypersensitive, gives rise to referred pain and tenderness, and sometimes to referred autonomic phenomena and distortion of proprioception. Types include myofascial, cutaneous, fascial, ligamentous and periosteal trigger points. (p. 4)

Ischemic compression applied directly to the trigger point is an effective manual technique to deactivate TrPs. Other useful techniques for deactivating TrPs include muscle stripping, kneading, and stretching. (Also see Trigger Point Therapy in chapter 2.)

General Relaxation

General relaxation is a primary effect of massage that has many important benefits for athletes. When massage activates the parasympathetic nervous system, a person experiences the relaxation response, a complex phenomenon with multiple effects.

Important physiological and psychological aspects of the relaxation response include decreased oxygen consumption and metabolic rate; less strain on energy resources; increased intensity and frequency of alpha brain waves associated with deep relaxation; reduced blood lactates and blood substances associated with anxiety; significantly decreased blood pressure in people with hypertension; reduced heart rate and slower respiration; decreased muscle tension; increased blood flow to internal organs; decreased anxiety, fear, and phobias, and increased positive mental health; and improved quality of sleep (Robbins, Powers, & Burgess, 1994).

The relaxation response is a mind–body phenomenon. It can be induced either by calming the mind first, followed by physiological effects (i.e., psychosomatic), or by relaxing the body first, followed by psychological effects (i.e., somatopsychic). The various effects are so interrelated that inducing one will tend to reflexively set off the others. For example, deep, slow breathing is commonly used to induce the relaxation response. Muscle relaxation can have the same effect and is especially effective when supplemented by diaphragmatic breathing.

The slow, smooth, sliding movements of massage activate the parasympathetic nervous system and trigger the relaxation response. It should come as no surprise that massage is particularly relaxing when performed on the back (Field et al., 1992; Yates, 2004).

Anxiety Reduction

Anxiety (i.e., worrying and uneasiness of mind) can distract athletes, causing lapses of concentration and focus. If it lasts for a long period of time, anxiety adds to the overall stress experienced by athletes.

Anxiety reduction is a consistent finding in studies on the effects of massage. This can benefit athletes who are training hard and preparing for important competitive events, as well as those feeling stress from other life circumstances.

Although we often think of anxiety as a mental phenomenon, it is actually emotional with both mind and body components. Anxiety is measured in research studies through self-reporting instruments, and also using objective measures of cortisol levels in saliva and urine. Anxiety reduction is one of the effects of the relaxation response discussed previously. It may also be related to the release of endorphins as a result of massage (Field, 2000; Kaard & Tostinbo, 1989; Rich, 2002).

Anxiety-reducing massage consists of sliding, kneading, and other techniques applied in a calm, smooth, relaxing manner. Stimulating techniques such as percussion and techniques that cause pain should be avoided.

Feelings of Well-Being

A positive outlook on life and general feelings of well-being offer a solid emotional base for the athlete. Massage given to a variety of populations experiencing stress has been shown to elevate mood and to alleviate depression. This is true at all life stages from children, to adolescents, to seniors. This overall effect is the result of reduced stress, reduced anxiety, and the release of endorphins, which are natural mood elevators (Field, 2000; Rich, 2002).

Increased Mental Alertness and Clarity

Mental alertness and clarity of mind are important readiness factors for competition, concentrating on learning a new skill, or perfecting the details of a difficult move. Massage performed at a fast pace using stimulating techniques has been found to increase mental acuity.

In a job stress study conducted in 1993, subjects received a 20-minute massage in a chair twice weekly for a month. They reported less fatigue and demonstrated greater clarity of thought, improved cognitive skills, and lower anxiety levels. Measurements such as EEG and alpha, beta, and theta brain waves showed alterations consistent with improved alertness (Field, 2000; Field, Fox, Pickens, Ironsong, & Scafidi, 1993).

Increased mental acuity is related to sensory stimulation and increased circulation to the brain. Improved mental clarity may also be the result of a calmer mind. Research suggests that short massage sessions (10 to 15 minutes), with an upbeat tempo, and using stimulating techniques such as percussion and passive joint mobilizing, improve mental sharpness.

Secondary Effects

The secondary effects of sports massage are performance-related outcomes of the primary effects. For example, the prevention and breaking of tissue adhesions (primary) lead to more pain-free and fluid muscle movements (secondary), which are essential for quality performance. Improved blood circulation (primary) promotes faster recovery from heavy workouts (secondary), which permits more frequent and concentrated practice sessions leading to a more polished performance. Following are some of the important secondary effects of massage.

Greater Energy

Energy is depleted and fatigue sets in when the body cannot keep up with supplying nutrients and carrying away waste products from muscles in continuous contraction. Muscular contractions occur consciously from movement and also unconsciously, such as with chronically hypertonic muscles or those in spasm. Chronically tight muscles may be the result of inadequate recovery or of a sustained stress response.

Massage helps in an active way by improving circulation, which hastens the removal of metabolites and makes the nutrients needed for muscle relaxation more available. Massage also prevents energy depletion through both muscular and general relaxation. The athlete, therefore, has more energy for training and competition.

Freer Movement at Joints

A number of soft tissue conditions can restrict movement at a joint. These include hypertonic muscles, scarring in muscle and connective tissue, adhesions, trigger points, and connective tissue shortening and rigidity. Application of appropriate massage techniques alleviates these conditions and allows a normal range of movement. The same factors that inhibit range of motion also affect the ability of the athlete to move smoothly and gracefully.

A cooperative study by sport physical therapists and a massage therapist found that massage can significantly increase range of motion in the hamstrings (Crosman, Chateauvert, & Weisburg, 1985). Increased flexibility was immediately evident and lasted for at least seven days postmassage. The massage techniques used were light, deep, and stretching effleurage (sliding strokes); petrissage (kneading); and deep circular and transverse friction.

Faster Recovery

Athletes require adequate time to recover from intense training and competition. Recovery is an essential, although often ignored, aspect of training. The accumulation of negative effects results in overtraining syndrome, which is characterized by increased frequency of injury, irritability, increased resting heart rate, altered appetite, apathy, and decreased quality of performance (Anshel, 1991).

Sports massage addresses many aspects of recovery, including the reduction of muscle soreness and stiffness caused by accumulated metabolites, the acceleration of tissue repair, the relaxation and lengthening of tight muscles, and general relaxation to restore physical and emotional balance. Zalessky (1979) summarized the restorative effects of massage in his article "Coaching, Medico-Biological and Psychological Means of Restoration."

> Under the influence of massage, blood circulation is improved; removal of wastes and toxic substances from tissues is accelerated; metabolic and oxidative processes are activated; central and peripheral nervous system activity is normalized. Massage accelerates resorption of infiltrates in muscles, ligaments, and tendons; decreases muscle tension after work; increases functional neuromuscular activity.

Greater Work Capacity.   A historic study on recovery massage done by Mosso and Maggiora at the turn of the 20th century focused on restoring work capacity in muscles. R. Tait McKenzie reported in 1915 that "there was a greater increase in working capacity after the use of petrissage [kneading] than from either of the other movements [friction and percussion], but the best results were obtained by using in turn all three [techniques]" (pp. 338-339).

This early research on the effects of massage to increase work capacity was substantiated in a 1990 study by Jordan and Jessup at the University of North Carolina at Chapel Hill, in which subjects performed a series of leg extensions on a Universal machine at 80 percent maximum until they could not continue (i.e., to extreme fatigue). The control group had passive rest after the leg extensions, and the experimental group received a 10-minute massage.

The study compared pretest and posttest torque readings of right quadriceps strength as measured by an isokinetic dynamometer. In the control group, strength decreased significantly, and in the experimental group, strength actually increased somewhat. The recovery massage given consisted of light and deep effleurage (sliding strokes), petrissage (kneading), and a compression broadening technique (Jordon & Jessup, 1990).

The early Mosso and Maggiora study traced the source of the recovery effects to improved circulation in the fatigued muscle (McKenzie, 1915). These findings were further confirmed in a more recent study of Russian athletes (Dubrovsky, 1982).

Massage, Exercise, and Rest.   McSwain (1990) compared the effects of massage, exercise, and rest on recovery after strenuous exercise by measuring the clearance rate of blood lactate. After a bout of strenuous exercise and a 5-minute interval, subjects were given either a 25-minute recovery massage (mainly sliding strokes and kneading), a 25-minute recovery exercise routine, or simply a rest period. Blood lactate levels (BLA) were measured at 5, 15, 30, and 50 minutes after the initial exercise.

As expected, both exercise and massage were more effective than rest for recovery. Massage and exercise were found to be equally effective (i.e., no statistically significant difference) during the period in which they were administered. However, the effects of massage were found to continue at a greater rate than the effects of exercise after treatment, and the massage group had the greatest percent decrease in BLA at the end of the 50-minute recovery period. Unfortunately, measurements were not taken after 50 minutes to see how long the effects of massage in decreasing BLA levels would have continued.

Based on her findings and a recommendation by Bell (1964), McSwain (1990) suggested that "a combination of exercise recovery (early in recovery), followed by massage (later during recovery) might be more effective in lowering BLA concentrations than either method of recovery alone" (p. 53). An alternative interpretation from McSwain's recovery period chart might be that if an athlete has at least 50 minutes between events, a 25-minute massage is more effective than exercise for recovery.

Combination of Recovery Methods.   A number of Russian studies supported the use of a combination of methods for recovery, given the time and resources. The Russians use a greater variety of recovery methods that include, in addition to exercise and massage, hydrotherapy (e.g., baths, sauna, steam room) and some physiotherapy methods (e.g., ultraviolet light, ultrasound, and electrotherapeutic procedures). All of these methods promote increased circulation and muscular and general relaxation (Birukov & Pogosyan, 1983; Matveeva & Tsirgiladze, 1985; Sinyakov & Belov, 1982; Zalessky, 1979).

Psychological Recovery.   Russian literature also discusses athletes' need to return to a normal psychological and emotional state following the stress of strenuous training and competition. What they call the "psychological means" of restoration include some familiar stress reduction and relaxation techniques termed psychoregulatory training (PRT)—for example, biofeedback and autogenic relaxation techniques. One article also mentioned such things as lifestyle and leisure time, a friendly team atmosphere, and even selecting music and colors to help achieve psychological recovery (Zalessky, 1979, 1980).

It is interesting that Russian literature does not mention massage as a means to general relaxation and stress reduction. Perhaps this is the result of their emphasis on the medical and physiological applications of massage. However, ample research supports the use of massage for psychological recovery (see the sections on general relaxation and anxiety reduction).

Pain Reduction

The pain reduction (analgesic) effect of massage is well documented (Kresge, 1983; Yates, 2004; Field, 2000). Because pain (i.e., the sensation of discomfort, distress, or suffering as a result of the irritation of pain sensors) is a complex phenomenon with many causal factors, the mechanisms for reducing pain using massage are also varied. These mechanisms include muscle relaxation and improved circulation, the deactivation of trigger points, the release of endorphins and serotonin, the gate theory, and the promotion of restorative sleep.

For example, muscle relaxation and improved circulation help relieve the pain associated with hypertonicity and the accompanying ischemia. A pain-spasm-pain cycle caused by muscular tension can be interrupted with application of massage (Kresge, 1983; Yates, 2004). And massage and stretching can relieve the pain associated with myofascial trigger points. This includes pain at the site of the TrP, satellite TrPs, and muscles that lie within the zone of reference of the TrP (Travell & Simons, 1983, 1992).

Evidence suggests that massage causes a release of central nervous system endorphins that modulate pain-impulse transmission. This may be the result of either physical or psychological effects of massage, and more research is needed to fully understand this mechanism (Yates, 2004).

In addition, several studies have found increased serotonin levels after massage therapy. Because serotonergic drugs are known to alleviate pain, the body's naturally produced serotonin could also be a pain reducer (Field, 2000).

Pain alleviation is also attributed to the gate theory (Melzack & Wall, 1965). According to this theory, pressure and cold stimuli are received in the spinal cord faster than pain impulses, and thereby close the neural gate on pain. So, by applying pressure to a site via massage, the related pain impulses are not processed. The neural-gating mechanism has been suggested as an explanation for the temporary analgesia associated with deep friction massage in the treatment of tendon and ligament injuries (Yates, 2004).

Finally, some researchers believe that massage may help reduce pain by promoting restorative sleep. During deep sleep, somatostatin, a chemical associated with pain reduction, is released. With sleep deprivation, Substance P, which is related to increased pain, is released. So, a person not getting enough sleep has decreased pain reduction capability and increased pain-producing substances. To the extent that relaxation massage promotes restful sleep, it contributes to pain reduction (Field, 2000).

Appropriate Level of Emotional Stimulation

An appropriate level of emotional stimulation is essential for peak performance. Low levels of stimulation leave an athlete feeling heavy, sluggish, or sleepy. High levels of stimulation can lead to feeling jumpy, distracted, or anxious. Either state impedes performance.

Applications of massage can be modified to help athletes achieve their optimal level of stimulation. Slow, smooth, relaxing massage with a lot of sliding strokes has an overall sedative effect that calms an athlete. On the other hand, upbeat, rigorous, fast-paced massage with kneading, squeezing, and percussion has an energizing and vitalizing effect (Birukov & Peisahov, 1979).

More Positive Outlook and Motivation

A negative outlook on life can diminish motivation to train hard and perform well. Because massage helps alleviate factors that sap positive feelings (e.g., pain, stress, and anxiety) and releases natural mood elevators (i.e., endorphins), it promotes a more positive outlook in athletes. The more intangible effects of caring touch and of encouraging words given by massage practitioners no doubt also have a positive effect on athletes receiving massage.

CONTRAINDICATIONS AND CAUTIONS

Sports massage should be avoided in all cases in which its application will worsen problem conditions. However, the concept of contraindication is not clearly defined. Most problem conditions are not absolute contraindications for massage, but certain cautions may be in order.

As a general rule, massage is contraindicated and should not be applied in the following situations:

- Around an infection
- Near suspected fractures
- Directly over open wounds or burns
- Near undiagnosed tumors
- Over varicose veins (avoid deep pressure)
- Where blood clots are present or suspected (e.g., phlebitis)
- Over a skin rash
- When contagious disease may be transmitted to the massage practitioners or to the athlete
- When an athlete is in severe distress (e.g., is nauseated, is in severe pain, or has a fever)

Caution applies for athletes with diabetes, kidney disease, cancer, and certain cardiac conditions, such as recent heart attack and excessively high or low blood pressure. In these cases, the athlete's health care provider should be contacted for any specific directions.

Caution is also in order for persons with cold and flu symptoms, as well as those reporting "not feeling well." Massage may worsen such conditions and cause nausea. During postevent sessions massage practitioners should watch for signs of dehydration and hyperthermia or hypothermia. They should not attempt sports massage until these conditions have subsided.

Extra caution should be taken during remedial applications of sports massage (e.g., with edema, strains, sprains, and tendinitis). Massage practitioners should not hesitate to refer the athlete for medical assessment when there is any doubt of the severity of a condition.

Severe inflammation is normally a contraindication for massage. However, experienced massage practitioners under medical supervision have applied massage as part of an overall treatment plan for inflamed tissues and joints. This situation calls for close monitoring and involves inflammation-reducing modalities and medication as part of the treatment plan. It is common practice for sports massage specialists to apply massage to conditions with associated mild inflammation.

Practitioners should take care to choose appropriate techniques and apply them correctly for the situation at hand. A condition may be worsened by one massage technique or approach but may respond positively to a different one. To apply massage safely and effectively, the practitioner should know the effects of each technique and its correct application. Further information on specific pathologies and their implications for massage can be found in special texts on the subject (see Rattray & Ludwig, 2000; Werner, 2002).

MEDICATIONS AND DRUGS

Massage practitioners should be aware of any medications an athlete is taking and their implications for sports massage. These include drugs for pain and inflammation, for managing emotional disorders, and for treating diseases such as diabetes and cardiovascular disease. Performance enhancers are an additional consideration.

Pain and Inflammation

Medications for pain (i.e., analgesics) include nonsteroidal anti-inflammatory drugs (NSAIDs), narcotic analgesics, skeletal muscle relaxants, and corticosteroids. Because of the physically demanding nature of sports, athletes are likely to use these medications at one time or another.

The most common NSAIDs taken for minor to moderate pain are aspirin and acetaminophen, which also have anticoagulant properties. Beware that athletes taking NSAIDs are more susceptible to bruising from massage techniques that use heavy pressure or that compress small spots (e.g., single-digit pressure). Also of concern is the effect of NSAIDs on feedback from the athlete. Because inflammation is reduced, an athlete may feel that his injury is further along in the healing process than the actual condition of the tissue warrants. In this case, the massage specialist should rely more on her palpation skills to assess the tissue condition and not be lured into working the tissues too aggressively.

Narcotic analgesics or opiates are taken for severe pain and have potential for physical dependence. Narcotic analgesics include morphine, hydrocodone, and codeine. These drugs depress nerve responses. In addition to the cautions about unreliable feedback, stretching techniques should be avoided or applied very carefully.

Muscle relaxants are taken for muscle spasm and spasticity. Muscles in athletes taking muscle relaxants will feel hypotonic and will not respond protectively to heavy pressure and overstretching. The massage specialist should lighten pressure and avoid stretches or keep stretches well within an easy range.

Corticosteroids are used to reduce immune or inflammatory response in conditions such as arthritis, tendinitis, bursitis, allergies, dermatological disorders, gastrointestinal diseases, and respiratory disorders such as asthma. Long-term use of these drugs can impair muscle strength, compromise tissue integrity, and reduce sensitivity. Body tissues in athletes using corticosteroids are more easily damaged by pressure and stretching. Techniques that stress musculoskeletal structures should be avoided or modified in these athletes (Persad, 2001).

Emotional Disorders

Medications for mood and emotional conditions (i.e., affective disorders) include anti-anxiety medications, antidepressants, and antipsychotic drugs. The first two categories of medications are being prescribed increasingly among the general population, including athletes.

Anti-anxiety medications are given for panic disorder, obsessive-compulsive behavior, post-traumatic stress disorder (PTSD), phobias, and generalized anxiety disorder. Antidepressants are prescribed for conditions such as major depression, bipolar depression, seasonal affective disorder, postpartum depression, and pain-induced depression. Antipsychotic drugs are given for major psychotic disorders such as schizophrenia.

Medications for emotional disorders vary in their effects on the body and mind, and in their potential side effects. Typical side effects for these types of medications include headaches and muscle and joint pain, which may not respond positively to massage. Other side effects such as dizziness, drowsiness, and lightheadedness may be heightened with massage. Massage practitioners should familiarize themselves with the side effects of clients' medications to better distinguish between the effects of massage and side effects of the drugs, and to identify contraindications.

Some medications for emotional disorders increase stress on the heart and cardiovascular system. Changes in sensory sensitivity and response to pain are common. Care should be taken to prevent stress on the body's systems and bruising.

For clients taking medications for emotional disorders, massage practitioners should provide a calming and safe environment and avoid techniques that are deep and aggressive. The overall effect of massage should be nurturing and relaxing (Persad, 2001).

Treatment of Diseases

Although athletes tend to be healthier than the average person, many suffer from some disease. Modern medicine and knowledge of disease processes have allowed athletes who in times past would have hung up their playing shoes to continue to train and compete. Moreover, people are participating in sport activities all through the life span into their senior years.

The sports massage specialist should be familiar with common diseases and their implications for massage. Although it is not in the scope of this text to review all possible diseases, two common diseases are discussed in the following sections: diabetes and cardiovascular disease.

Diabetes

Diabetes is a disorder of carbohydrate metabolism. Athletes with diabetes may take insulin to control blood sugar levels, or in mild cases may rely on diet.

Diabetes eventually results in deterioration of cardiovascular and connective tissues and loss of feeling, especially in the extremities. Tissue healing is slow and poor. In advanced cases, tissues may be fragile and easily damaged. People with diabetes are more susceptible to infection. Pressure on damaged tissues should be light, and sessions should be shortened as necessary to avoid instability (i.e., dangerous fluctuations of blood sugar levels).

Stability of blood sugar is a major concern in people with diabetes because instability can be life threatening. If possible, those with diabetes should schedule massages for times when their blood sugar is most likely to be stable. This varies from person to person. Practitioners should avoid massaging directly over the site of a recent insulin injection. They should be prepared to respond to an episode of instability to avoid insulin shock. For first aid for diabetic instability, always give sugar (e.g., candy, fruit, sugar); never give insulin.

Cardiovascular Disease

Cardiovascular (CV) disease will be an increasing concern in sports massage as more senior athletes remain active. Common cardiovascular diseases include high blood pressure (hypertension), hardening of the arteries (atherosclerosis), chest pain (angina pectoris), heart attack, uneven heart rhythm (cardiac dysrhythmia), and stroke.

Medications for cardiovascular conditions include those that improve heart function, increase blood vessel diameter, alter blood coagulation mechanisms, reduce blood volume (diuretics), and lower blood lipid levels. Practitioners should know all of their clients' heart medications and their effects on the body, including undesirable side effects.

Examples of massage considerations related to CV medications include lightening pressure on athletes taking anticoagulants, anticipating dizziness and lightheadedness in those taking drugs for hypertension, avoiding injection sites, and using side-lying or seated position for those unable to lie supine. Some CV medications make people more prone to contraindications such as deep-vein thrombosis. Practitioners should monitor athletes taking CV medications carefully for adverse side effects and refer them for medical attention as needed.

The subject of massage therapy and medications is an extensive one that deserves the attention of the sports massage specialist. For information on specific medications, consult a current reference on prescription drugs. *Massage Therapy & Medications* by Persad (2001) offers an overview of medications and their implications for massage therapy.

Performance-Enhancing Drugs

The use of drugs to unfairly enhance performance is a serious issue at all levels of sport. The United States Anti-Doping Agency has identified prohibited classes of drugs. These include stimulants, narcotics, anabolic steroids, peptide hormones, beta-2 agonists, agents with anti-estrogen activity, and masking agents. For more information, visit their Web site at www.usantidoping.org.

Doping presents a special problem to massage practitioners because many of these drugs have adverse side effects that are contraindications for massage. This is especially true of drugs that alter cardiovascular function and damage tissue integrity. If doping is suspected, sports massage specialists should discuss the situation with the coach or the physician heading the health care support team.

Chapter 2 describes in detail the basic techniques used in sports massage, identifies the effects of each technique, and makes suggestions for their use with athletes.

STUDY QUESTIONS

1. What are the five major applications of sports massage?
2. How do sports massage specialists enhance athletic performance?
3. What is meant by the "whole athlete," and why is this concept important for understanding the factors that affect success in sports?
4. In what ways does sports massage increase an athlete's performance potential?
5. How does the "magic bullet" contrast with the "cumulative effects" explanation for the effectiveness of sports massage?
6. What is the constellation of effects theory of sports massage? Give examples of chain reactions of primary and secondary effects.
7. What are the important physical factors in athletic performance, and how can massage contribute to their improvement?
8. How do psychological factors affect athletic performance, and how can massage contribute to their improvement?
9. When is sports massage contraindicated, and what cautions should be observed when giving massage to athletes?
10. What are the cautions related to medications/drugs and massage?

TECHNIQUES AND BASIC SKILLS

LEARNING OUTCOMES

1. Describe basic hand and finger positions for performing massage techniques.
2. Identify eight basic sports massage techniques and explain their effects.
3. Describe the application of massage techniques with active movement.
4. List the categories of joint movement techniques and give examples.
5. Describe specialized massage techniques and their uses in sports massage.
6. Understand the value of palpation skills in sports massage.

BUILDING BLOCKS OF SPORTS MASSAGE

Individual massage techniques are the building blocks of a sports massage session. Skilled practitioners combine these techniques into therapeutic sequences and perform them with the rhythm, pace, and pressure needed to produce the desired results. Sports massage practitioners must understand the physiological and psychological effects of techniques and their combinations to apply them effectively.

The massage techniques presented here are manual techniques except for the use of vibration devices. The human hand can be a very precise instrument. It is capable of sensing myriad bits of information about the condition of the tissues it is touching and of performing techniques with finely coordinated movements. The information in this chapter provides a knowledge base for thoughtful and informed practice of the manual techniques of sports massage.

The techniques described in this chapter are largely derived from Western massage and are the basis for most sports massage performed in North America and Europe today. Specialized techniques such as positional release, trigger point therapy, myofascial massage, and lymphatic drainage massage are also integrated into sports massage sessions. These specialized techniques have therapeutic goals targeted toward specific tissues and body systems and will be discussed briefly at the end of this chapter.

HAND AND FINGER POSITIONS

For a clear understanding of how to apply massage techniques, it is essential to consider basic hand positions and finger placements. These fundamental positions are used to apply the techniques described later in the chapter.

Single-Digit Placement

In *single-digit placement*, the tip or pad of a single finger or the thumb applies the massage technique. The rest of the hand may touch the athlete, but the massage movement comes from a single digit. Figure 2.1 demonstrates the use of single-digit placement for applying pressure to muscle attachments, in this case those associated with tennis elbow. It is especially useful in self-massage.

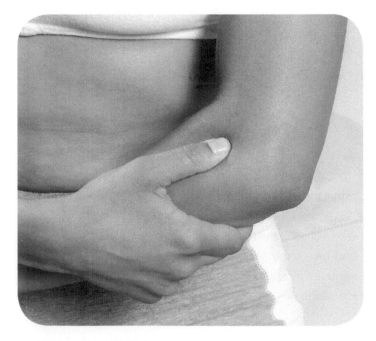

Figure 2.1   Single-digit placement.

Single-Digit Overlay

Single-digit overlay involves single-digit placement supported by the use of another digit of the same or the other hand. One finger applies the massage while the other is placed on top to assist with strength and coordination of the massage movement (see figure 2.2).

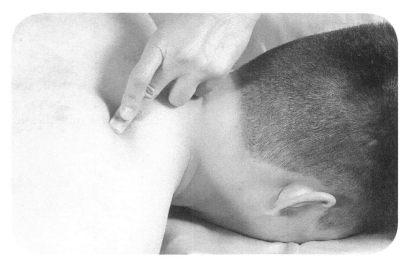

Figure 2.2 Single-digit overlay.

Multiple-Digit Placement

In multiple-digit placement, the tips or the pads of several fingers or both thumbs apply the massage. Figure 2.3 demonstrates the effective use of multiple-digit placement for sliding movements over the length of a muscle. It is especially effective for hard-to-reach places such as the back of the neck.

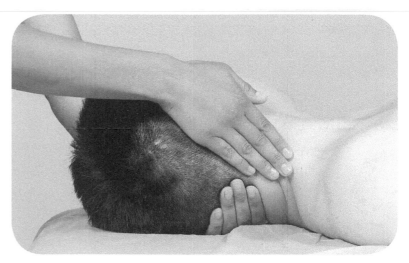

Figure 2.3 Multiple-digit placement.

Multiple-Digit Overlay

In multiple-digit overlay, the fingers of one hand apply the technique while the fingers of the other hand are placed on top of the first to assist with strength and coordination of the massage movement (see figure 2.4).

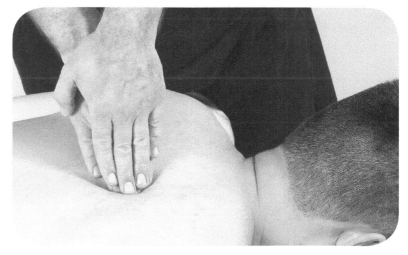

Figure 2.4 Multiple-digit overlay.

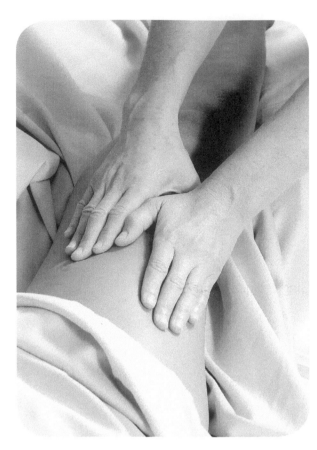

Figure 2.5 Full-palmar placement.

Full-Palmar Placement

For full-palmar placement, the entire palmar surface of one hand or both hands, including the digits, is in contact with the surface to be massaged (see figure 2.5). This broad contact is useful for techniques intended to move fluids, such as sliding techniques used to increase circulation.

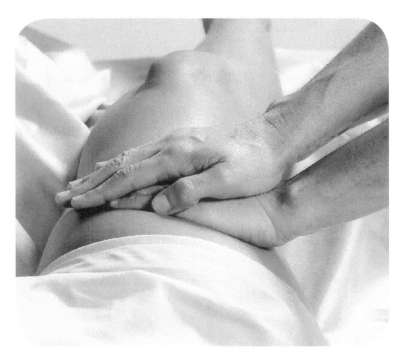

Figure 2.6 Full-palmar overlay.

Full-Palmar Overlay

In full-palmar overlay, the entire palmar surface of one hand applies the massage technique while the palm of the other hand is placed on top to assist with strength and coordination of the movement. This placement is especially useful for applying more pressure when working on large, well-muscled areas. Figure 2.6 shows full-palmar overlay used to reinforce the bottom hand when performing compression to the thigh muscles.

Knuckle Placement

The dorsal surface of the proximal phalanx bones performs the massage when the hands are in knuckle placement. The entire length of the bones makes contact, not just the knobby joints. This placement is not performed with a tight fist, which is rigid and unyielding, but with an open fist, which allows for some resilience when pressure is applied. Figure 2.7 shows the contact surface in proper knuckle placement.

Fist Placement

Fist placement is similar to knuckle placement except that the fingers are closed into a fist. For massage, the fist is held loosely; the contact surface for applying the technique is the same as in knuckle placement. The fist is used to apply deep pressure to large muscles such as the gluteals. It is used for sliding and compression techniques.

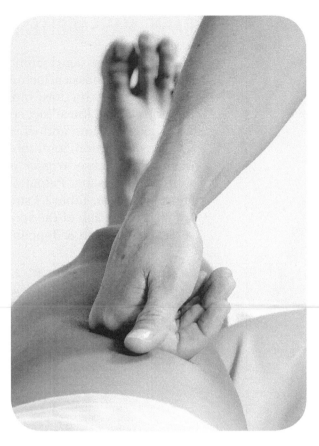

Figure 2.7 Knuckle placement.

Forearm Placement

The forearm can be used to apply deep pressure to broad surfaces such as the back and the thigh. The elbow is bent, and pressure is applied with the flat ulnar surface. Use of the forearm can reduce wear and tear on the practitioner's hands. Figure 2.8 shows sliding applied to the back using the forearm.

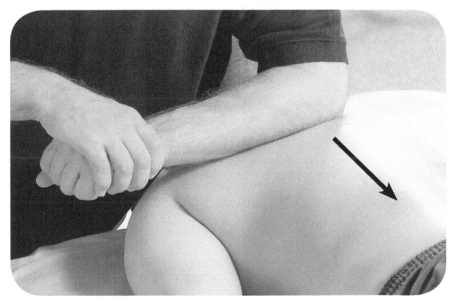

Figure 2.8 Sliding movement on the back using the forearm.

BASIC MASSAGE TECHNIQUES

Most sports massage techniques are derived from traditional Western massage. Although any massage technique can be integrated into a sports massage session, this text focuses on those most commonly used. Basic sports massage techniques include sliding, kneading, compression, skin lifting, percussion, superficial friction, deep friction, and vibration. Joint movement techniques include range of motion evaluation, joint mobilizing, and stretching. Specialized techniques are positional release, trigger point therapy, myofascial massage, and lymphatic drainage massage. Palpation skills are essential to the skillful application of sports massage. Table 2.1 summarizes the primary physiological and psychological effects of each of the sports massage techniques described in this text. (Also refer to Benjamin & Tappan, 2005.)

Table 2.1 Effects of Sports Massage Techniques

Technique	Effects
Palmar sliding	Move fluids Sooth nervous system Stretch and compress soft tissues
Faltering effleurage	Stimulate nerve receptors
Thumb slides	Broaden soft tissues Stretch specific muscle tissue Reduce muscle tension
Broadening	Broaden and separate muscle tissue
Kneading	Warm soft tissues Increase local circulation Increase tissue pliability Relax muscles
Palmar compression (pumping)	Increase circulation Increase tissue pliability Broaden muscles
Palmar compression (sustained)	Reduce muscle tension or spasm
Palmar compression (rocking)	Create joint movement Increase circulation
Digital compression	Hold tender points for positional release Deactivate trigger points (ischemic compression) Press stress points Stimulate acu-points

Technique	Effects
Skin lifting/rolling	Separate fascial tissues
	Increase local circulation
Percussion	Stimulate nerve endings
	Increase mental clarity and alertness
	Improve mental focus
Superficial friction	Warm tissues
	Increase local circulation
	Stimulate nerve endings
Deep circular friction	Manipulate soft tissues around joints
	Increase soft tissue pliability
Deep transverse friction	Break fascial adhesions
	Treat tendinitis
	Form healthy scar tissue
Vibration	Stimulate physiological processes
	Increase local circulation
	Relax muscles
	Reduce pain

Sliding

Sliding is performed by moving the hand on the skin from one place to another applying steady pressure. Sliding is usually done using oil or lotion to reduce friction and irritation. Sliding movements are very effective and easy to learn and have many variations and uses.

Basic Sliding

Figure 2.9 depicts the most common type of sliding movement using full-palmar placement. The hands remain relaxed and conform to the body surface throughout the entire movement. Using steady pressure, a long sliding motion is performed along the length of the part to be massaged. Pressure is lightened over bony prominences such as the elbow or patella. Upon completion of the sliding movement in one direction, the hands move back to the starting point by sliding superficially over the skin surface. Pressure on the return movement is only enough to maintain contact.

Variations of the basic sliding movement are achieved by simply changing the hand placement to any of those described earlier (e.g., single-digit, multiple-digit, knuckle, or fist placement, or by using the forearm). You can also vary the direction and the amount of pressure. With experience, you can create many effective variations of sliding.

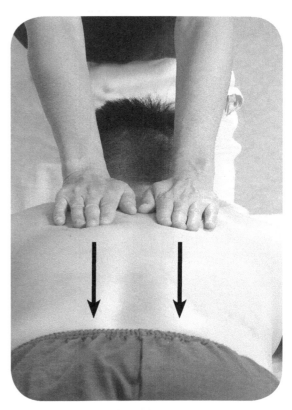

Figure 2.9 Basic sliding using full-palmar hand position.

Moving Fluids.   Sliding movements are effective at moving body fluids such as blood and lymph. They are used along with kneading in recovery applications to flush metabolites out of tissues after intense physical activity. They are also used to enhance circulation where injury or immobilization has restricted blood flow.

Sliding movements can benefit the healthy circulatory system by enhancing normal venous return. Sliding movements on the arms and legs are usually performed in the direction of the heart (i.e., distal to proximal) to prevent damage to valves in the veins. Sliding moves stale, low-oxygen blood out of an area and leaves room for its replacement with oxygen-rich blood.

Sliding movements also assist the flow of lymphatic fluid toward the lymph nodes where foreign substances are filtered out. This is especially important for tissue repair during recovery and rehabilitation.

Edema (i.e., abnormal accumulation of fluid in tissues) caused by poor local circulation, stress on joints, or recent injury may be reduced using sliding movements in the direction of lymph flow. Pressure should be light to avoid damaging tissues.

Athletes with a history of phlebitis or blood clots should not have their extremities massaged with heavy pressure, which could dislodge the clot. Also, any type of inflammation or edema caused by infection is a contraindication for circulatory massage, which might spread the infection. Athletes with cancer should check with their physicians before receiving massage that increases circulation.

Soothing the Nervous System.   Sliding techniques performed with light to moderate pressure in a slow, steady, rhythmical manner activate the parasympathetic nervous system. This produces the relaxation response discussed in chapter 1. The relaxation response is important in recovery applications of sports massage.

Sliding techniques performed with extremely light pressure can reduce neurosensitivity in situations of acute pain. For example, an athlete with a minor cervical injury may exhibit a great deal of associated muscle spasm, voluntary and involuntary splinting, and apprehension toward treatment. Sliding techniques performed over the area with very light pressure and in a steady, even rhythm can reduce neurosensitivity and will often elicit relaxation of the underlying muscles. Stress and anxiety are also reduced. As a result, the athlete may be more open to other forms of treatment.

Faltering Effleurage

Faltering effleurage is a combination sliding movement and superficial friction found in Russian-style massage. It is performed with little or no oil and has a warming and stimulating effect. In faltering effleurage, the hands alternate in short, swift, brushing slides over the skin as shown in figure 2.10. The hands are held stiffly, and the rhythm is uneven (i.e., stroke, stroke, pause). The fast pace, change in rhythm, and brisk movements stimulate nerve receptors in the skin.

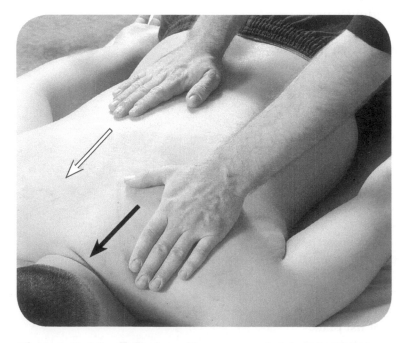

Figure 2.10   Faltering effleurage—a brisk movement that combines sliding and superficial friction for a stimulating effect.

Thumb Slides

Sliding the thumb along a specific muscle from attachment to attachment while applying heavy pressure is called a *thumb slide*. The distal segment, or thumb pad, is the contact point. The thumb should be positioned in a straight line with the radius of the lower arm to avoid damage to the thumb joints.

Thumb slides differ from the basic palmar sliding described earlier in that their effect is specific to the muscle involved; they have little effect on general circulation. Thumb slides are used to reduce muscle tension, increase muscle elasticity, and broaden and elongate muscle fibers. Thumb slides provide a slight spot-specific stretch, which makes them useful for areas difficult to stretch otherwise, such as the tibialis anterior on the front of the shin (see figure 2.11).

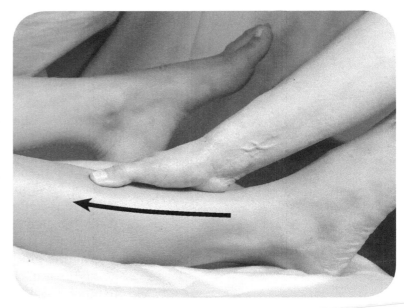

Figure 2.11 Thumb slide on tibialis anterior using single-digit placement.

Thumb slides to a single muscle are repeated several times for best effect. *Muscle stripping* involves performing thumb slides in parallel lines over the width of a muscle.

Broadening

Broadening refers to a sliding technique that first compresses muscle and fascial tissues followed by sliding in a direction transverse (i.e., perpendicular) to the length of the muscle fibers. This action broadens or separates the tissues. Broadening techniques can be applied to muscle bellies as well as to tendons.

For large muscles or muscle groups, the hands are positioned on the area in full-palmar placement, with the heels of the hands meeting in the center of the muscle (see figure 2.12). Sufficient pressure is applied with the heel of the hands to compress the tissues while the palms move out and away from one another in a direction transverse to the length of the muscle fibers. The movement is repeated along the length of the muscle group over the entire area.

Broadening on a small area such as the forearm is performed using the thumbs. Place the thumbs next to each other on the muscle to be broadened. Slide the thumbs away from each other, broadening the muscle tissue as shown in figure 2.13.

Broadening techniques help restore muscles to their optimal contraction potential, which is important for strength and power in sports. Muscle strength is related to its ability to contract (i.e., shorten and broaden). Hypertonic muscles feel hard and ropelike, especially

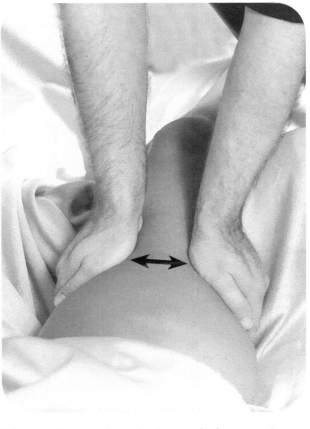

Figure 2.12 Broadening technique on the quadriceps using full-palmar placement.

in chronic conditions. They do not contract and relax optimally, and they suffer injury more easily. Broadening techniques help restore muscles to their natural broadening potential.

Kneading

In *kneading*, the hands alternately and rhythmically squeeze, lift, and release the muscle. Kneading is typically performed on groups of muscles rather than on individual muscles and is applied to the muscle bellies rather than to attachments.

Basic kneading begins with the hands in full-palmar position. When massaging larger muscle groups such as the quadriceps, use two-handed kneading as shown in figure 2.14. First, squeeze and lift with one hand and then the other in a rhythmical and alternating motion. Repeat this movement in different places along the muscle belly with a moderate tempo. Take care not to pinch the skin or adipose tissue. Adjust the pressure to avoid causing pain or bruising.

Use one-handed kneading to massage smaller muscle groups such as the extensors in the forearm. Figure 2.15 shows how to use one hand to support the arm while the other hand kneads the muscle belly.

When applying the technique, note the warming of tissues and the increasing muscle elasticity. Kneading produces passive muscle movement and a slight stretch. Local circulation is increased, and hypertonicity is reduced. Used as an evaluation method, kneading can help the massage practitioner determine the overall condition of any given muscle group.

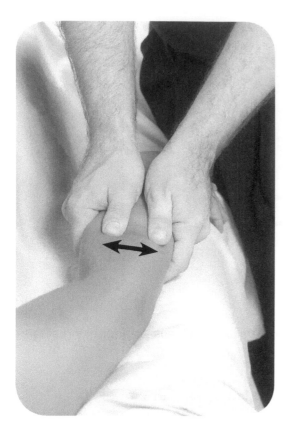

Figure 2.13 Broadening technique on the forearm using the thumbs.

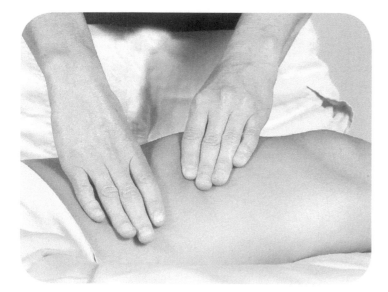

Figure 2.14 Kneading with two hands.

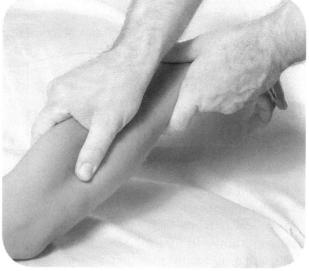

Figure 2.15 Using one hand for support while the other hand performs the kneading technique on the forearm.

Compression

In *compression* techniques, the tissues are compressed against surrounding soft tissues and bone. The most common types of compression used in sports massage are palmar compression and digital compression. Palmar compression techniques are used to increase local circulation, and digital compression techniques are used for different types of "point" or spot-specific applications.

Palmar Compression

Palmar compression is applied with the hands placed on the muscle group in the palmar overlay position as shown in figures 2.16 and 2.17. The area of contact for applying the technique is the palm and heel of the bottom hand with the fingers playing a lesser role. Note that the top hand is placed over the metacarpals of the bottom hand and *not* over the wrist. Pointing the fingers in the same direction will help keep wrists in a neutral position. Putting pressure on the wrist while performing compressions, or applying pressure while the wrist is hyperextended, can result in wrist injury.

Pressure is applied by shifting the body weight into the hands. This is done in a repeated rhythmic motion described as *pumping*. This straight-up-and-down motion presses the muscle tissues into each other and into the underlying bone (see figure 2.16).

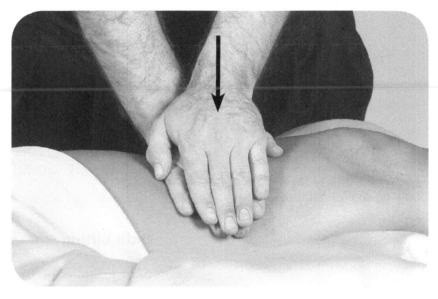

Figure 2.16 Palmar compression—pumping.

Palmar compression performed at a brisk pace creates *durable hyperemia* or blood flow to an area, and is a staple of pre-event massage. It warms the muscles and invigorates the athlete, increasing readiness for activity. Palmar compression applied more slowly and with a greater amount of pressure is used to reduce muscle tension or spasm, create a site-specific stretch or broadening of tissues, and increase elongation potential.

A variation called *rocking* is performed by pushing the tissues forward as compressions are applied, a "down and away" motion (see figure 2.17). This creates movement in surrounding joints that adds a kinesthetic dimension to the technique.

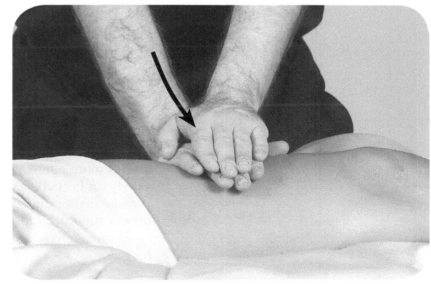

Figure 2.17 Rocking compression.

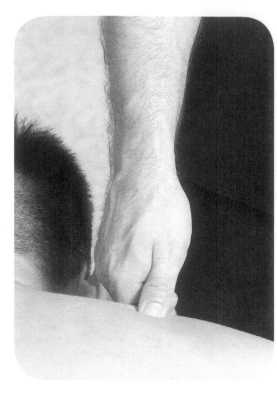

Figure 2.18 Wrist alignment for applying digital compression.

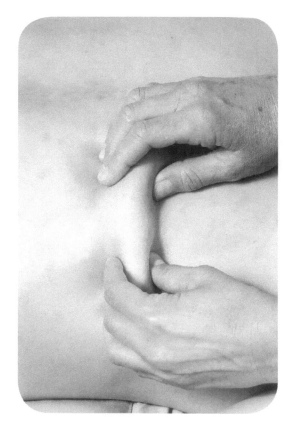

Figure 2.19 Skin rolling.

Digital Compression

Digital compression is a simple technique performed with the thumb, fingertips, or elbow. Pressure is applied with sufficient force to compress the tissues underneath. Digital compression may be applied to one point after another along a specific muscle, or as one prolonged application to a specific point.

When applying digital compression, keep the thumb or fingers in straight alignment with the wrist as shown in figure 2.18. The line of force is through the joints into the larger arm bones, and not across any joints. This straight alignment prevents injury to the joints involved in the technique application.

Digital compression has many uses in sports massage. A variation called *ischemic compression* is used to deactivate trigger points. Digital pressure with the thumb is used to hold points in strain–counterstrain and positional release techniques. "Stress points" in tendons and muscle are pressed using digital compression (Meagher, 1990; Travell & Simons, 1983, 1992).

Acu-points (i.e., energy points) are pressed using digital compression in bodywork systems such as acupressure and shiatsu. Practitioners trained in these systems may apply them in their work with athletes (Namikoshi, 1985; Nickle, 1984).

Skin Lifting

Skin lifting is performed by picking up the superficial skin layers and gently pulling them away from the underlying muscle tissue. There are a few different ways to move from one spot to another while covering a specific area. You can use two hands side by side to lift a greater area of skin, and then release and move them to a different spot. Or, you can alternate left and right hands moving from one spot to another. If the skin is loose (i.e., adhering less to underlying tissues), you can stay in contact and roll the skin along using the thumbs to push the skin up against the opposing fingers as shown in figure 2.19. This last technique is called *skin rolling*.

Before performing skin lifting or rolling, the whole area should be warmed with sliding, kneading, or compression techniques. This increases circulation in the area and makes tissues more pliable. Lifting and rolling should be performed slowly for best effects, and to prevent unnecessary pain.

Skin lifting and rolling increases local circulation and breaks superficial myofascial adhesions. It is used effectively to enhance circulation to generally tense areas such as the back.

Percussion

Percussion is the general term for a variety of techniques that apply rapid, rhythmic percussive movements to the body (see figure 2.20). The six common forms of percussion used in sports massage are beating, hacking, slapping, cupping, pincement, and tapping.

All variations of percussion are performed in a similar fashion, but different forms use different striking surfaces and create their own unique sound. The athlete feels a slightly different sensation from each variation, but the end result is the same—physical and mental stimulation.

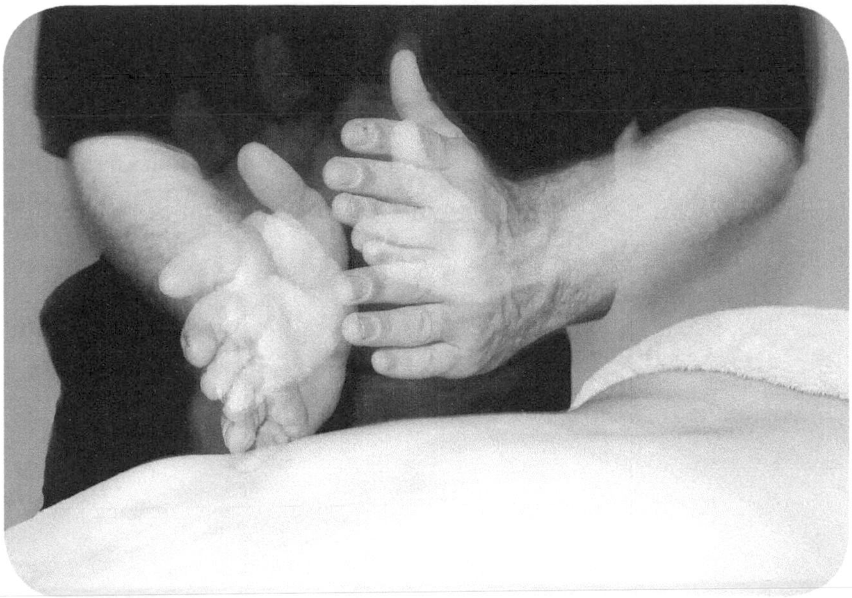

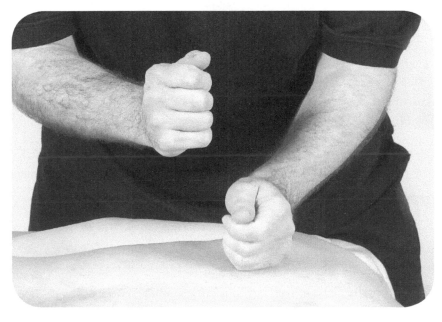

Figure 2.20   Rapid movement of percussion.

Percussion techniques should be performed with relaxed hands and fingers. Hands alternate hitting the body surface with light, rapid, rhythmic movements. The hands bounce off of the skin.

Percussion can be performed on any muscle group. The force used is modified for lighter and heavier muscled areas. Avoid hitting bony prominences, and do not perform percussion over organs that might be damaged from the technique (e.g., over the kidneys or in the abdominal area).

Percussion performed skillfully is pleasant and stimulating, enhancing an athlete's readiness for practice or competition. Different forms can be mixed for a very upbeat and invigorating effect.

Beating

In the form of percussion called *beating*, the hands are in a lightly closed fist. The slightly padded hypothenar eminence (side of the hand) and the little finger form the striking surface. The wrist is kept loose, rather than rigid, during the movement so that the effect is not jarring to the recipient. See figure 2.21.

Figure 2.21   Beating.

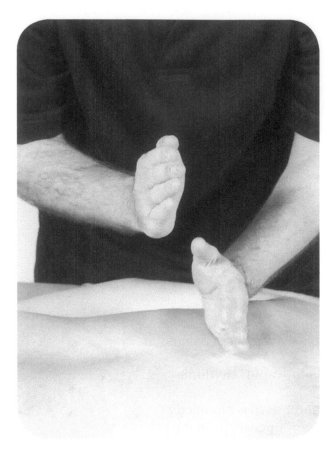

Figure 2.22 Hacking.

Hacking

In *hacking*, the hands are held with the palms facing each other, and the fingers are relaxed in slight flexion. The little (fifth) finger is more relaxed than the fourth; the fourth more relaxed than the third; and so on. The little finger and the tips of the fourth and third fingers form the main striking surface. The side of the hand (i.e., hypothenar eminence) may also hit lightly. The wrist and fingers remain loose during the movement. See figure 2.22.

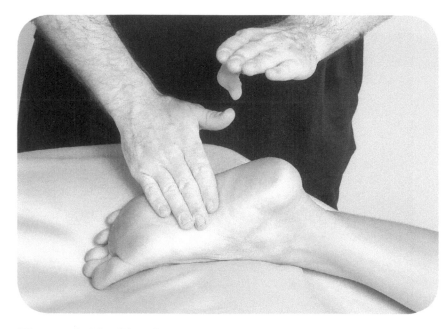

Figure 2.23 Slapping.

Slapping

In *slapping*, the hands are held with the palms facing the athlete's body. Use either the entire palmar surface or just the pads of the fingers to lightly slap the skin. See figure 2.23.

Cupping

In *cupping*, the hands are held so that the thumb and fingers are pressed together and slightly flexed with the palmar surface becoming concave and forming a cup. The striking surface is the outer rim of the "cup," formed by the little finger, fingertips, thumb, and heel of the hand (see figure 2.24). The center of the palm does not make contact. Cupping creates a hollow sound.

The action of cupping involves more than the striking surface hitting the skin. If performed skillfully, the "cup" creates a kind of vacuum, which some believe can loosen broad, flat areas of fascial adhesion. Cupping is also used for loosening congestion in the lungs and respiratory system.

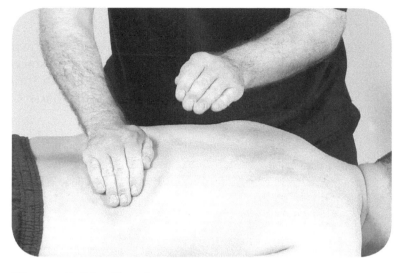

Figure 2.24   Cupping.

Pincement

In *pincement*, the hands are held with palms facing the athlete's body. The thumb and fingers are used to lightly pick up, or pluck, the superficial tissues (see figure 2.25). Perform pincement rapidly, but do not pinch the skin aggressively.

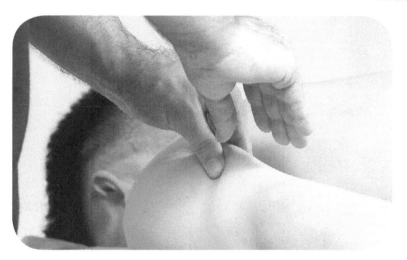

Figure 2.25   Pincement.

Tapping

In *tapping*, the fingertips or pads lightly tap the skin (see figure 2.26). This is the most delicate of the percussion techniques and is useful on the face, head, and chest.

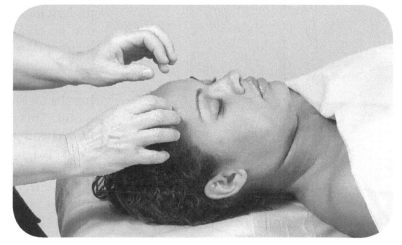

Figure 2.26   Tapping.

Friction

Friction is one of the oldest known massage techniques and has been mentioned in medical and health texts since ancient times. One trainer in the early 20th century remarked, "When in training after running and perspiring freely one should subject the skin to harsh friction from coarse towels" (Pollard, 1902).

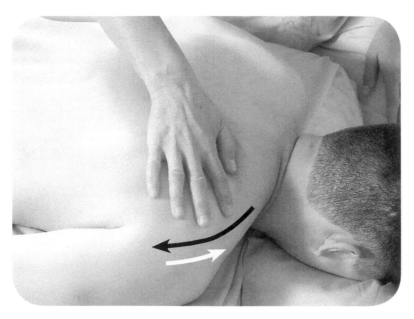

Figure 2.27 Superficial warming friction.

Superficial Friction

Superficial friction is stimulating and is used to increase superficial blood flow for a warming effect. For example, it is quite natural to rub your skin briskly when you feel cold.

Superficial friction can be performed using one of many different hand placements (e.g., the palmar surface of the hand, the knuckles, or the sides of the hands). The part used is moved rapidly back and forth over the surface of the skin, causing friction (see figure 2.27). The result is reddening and warming of the tissues.

Superficial friction was the essential technique of the athlete's rubdown, which preceded the more sophisticated movements of modern massage. It is a recommended form of self-massage with towels or brushes after a bath.

Deep Friction

Friction applied to deeper tissues is very specific in its application and is therefore performed with a small contact surface using the thumb, fingertips, or heel of the hand. The hand does not move over the surface of the skin as in superficial friction, but instead it moves the skin over the underlying tissues. If deeper pressure is used, movement can be created in a small spot on a structure such as a ligament, or it can move a band such as a tendon against surrounding tissues.

Sufficient pressure is applied so that the finger performing the technique and the skin it touches move together as a unit. This creates a friction effect on the tissues directly underneath as depicted in figure 2.28.

Deep friction warms the contact area and has the mechanical effect of breaking or reducing myofascial adhesions. Deep friction is applied to move tissues around joints, to massage tendons and ligaments, and to promote tissue healing and healthy scar formation. Two major types of deep friction are circular friction and deep transverse friction.

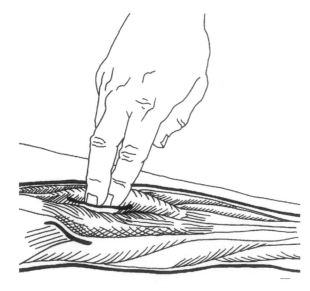

Figure 2.28 Deep friction affecting deeper tissues.

HISTORY BRIEF 3

The Rubdown

Athletes in the early 1900s were quite familiar with the rubdown, which consisted mainly of superficial friction with the hand or with objects such as a brush, horsehair glove, or coarse towel. In 1902 Pollard reported that

> Oxford athletes are never allowed to do cross country running without first rubbing their legs with horsehair gloves or with hands. . . . After sweating, sponge with hot saltwater. Dry with a coarse towel, then use a horsehair glove freely. . . . The best remedy for congestion and labored breathing is a glass of warm brandy and plenty of hard friction on the feet, legs and thighs. . . . In all cases vigorous rubbing should follow the use of water; a bath attendant who knows something about massage is invaluable, for how to rub down a man or a horse is an art. (p. 21)

Michael C. Murphy (1914), a well-known trainer and track coach, considered the rubdown a must for athletes. He advocated self-massage after a bath and advised that the back could be reached "with a rough towel" drawn back and forth vigorously. Murphy also used rubbing for sore shins. He said that "if the runner has the services of a trainer and rubber he will be properly cared for" (p. 161).

When more skilled massage became available, the rubdown fell out of favor. Matt Bullock at the University of Illinois wrote in 1925: "The beneficial effects of a good massage should not be confused with that anathema of the author—'rub down.' The conscientious trainer's language does not include the word, rub down, which is entirely too light and frivolous an expression of massage" (p. 15). *Rubdown* eventually came to mean a superficial, non-specific, low-skill massage.

Circular Friction. *Circular friction* is performed with a single digit, the fingertips, or the heels of the hands. The overlay placement may be used to generate greater force. Once enough pressure has been applied to move the skin, movement of the fingers or hands is in a circular pattern, counterclockwise or clockwise. The greater the pressure used, the deeper the underlying tissues that are affected. Figure 2.29 shows circular friction applied to the wrist.

Circular friction is useful around joints and on surfaces with little muscle such as the face and head, but it can be applied to any small area when affecting deeper tissues is desirable. It is used in sports massage for warming up joints prior to activity and is a useful technique for self-massage.

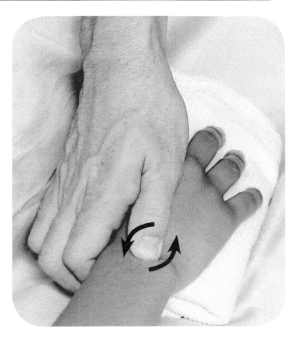

Figure 2.29 Deep circular friction moves skin over underlying tissues.

Deep Transverse Friction.   Because it is applied to very specific spots, *deep transverse friction* is performed with the pad of a reinforced finger (i.e. single-digit overlay) or thumb (see figure 3.7). The movement is back and forth across (i.e., transverse to) the direction of the muscle fibers, tendon, or ligament. Pressure is applied deep enough to affect the targeted tissues, and the skin moves with the finger.

Some believe that pain is an essential component of deep transverse friction. Pain seems to exist as long as unnecessary adhesions are present. The application of deep transverse friction becomes less painful as the adhesions break and tissues heal and become more mobile. Using techniques that cause pain should be done carefully, causing the least amount of pain necessary to reach the therapeutic goal. Refer to the section "Optimal Therapy Zone" in chapter 6.

Deep transverse friction is applied in the treatment of tendinitis and tenosynovitis, and is used to remove adhesions between tendons and ligaments, and in surrounding tissues.

Also known as Cyriax friction, it is used in rehabilitation to treat muscle and tendon lesions and to aid in the formation of healthy scar tissue.

Postinjury scars form in a haphazard manner with scar fibers overlapping one another in all directions. This healing process results in a matting effect in which muscle fibers adhere to each other and to surrounding connective tissue. A problem develops when extensive scarring limits the muscle's ability to contract and broaden. In addition, a site of chronic inflammation may develop where normal tissue joins scar tissue that is unable to accommodate changes in tension during muscle activity.

Deep transverse friction breaks adhesions between the scar tissue and surrounding fibers and leaves the scar itself intact. This process promotes the formation of a pliable, small scar that does not interfere with muscle contraction. It also reduces the potential for tearing at the site of the scar.

In the *Illustrated Manual of Orthopedic Medicine*, Cyriax and Cyriax (1993) presented some basic principles of using deep transverse friction to treat muscle and tendon lesions. These principles include the following:

○ Friction must be given deeply with the digit and skin moving together.

○ Administer friction to the precise site of the lesion.

○ The friction effect is most important, not the amount of pressure used.

○ Position the athlete to render the lesion accessible and to put the tissue being treated into appropriate tension.

○ A total of 6 to 12 sessions of 20 minutes each on alternate days is usually required for best results.

Sheathed tendons, such as the Achilles tendon, must be taut when applying deep transverse friction. This is to maximize the friction created between the sheath and the tendon itself.

Vibration

Vibration techniques are applied with a trembling motion in the fingertips or hand. Fingertips are typically placed in the multiple-digit overlay position, or the hand in full-palmar position resting lightly on the skin. The practitioner generates the trembling vibration with the shoulder, and from there it passes through the elbow to the hand and then to the tissues underneath (see figure 2.30).

Vibrations are applied in different single spots within a particular body region, or as an extended application while the hand slides along a section of the body. Light pressure affects superficial tissues, and deeper pressure affects deeper tissues.

Vibration increases local circulation and helps to relax muscles. Vibration is used to stimulate body processes (e.g., its use on the abdomen stimulates digestion and elimination). Vibration can soothe nervous tissue as in the treatment of peripheral neuritis. In cases of severe pain, light vibration may reduce pain impulses (see the discussion of the neural gating theory in chapter 1) so that other massage techniques can be applied.

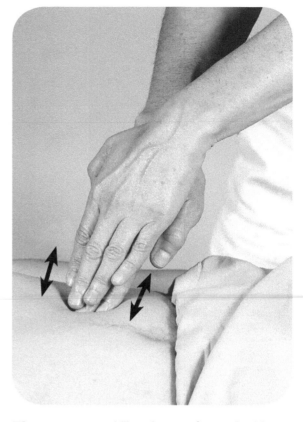

Figure 2.30 Vibration performed with multiple digits.

Use of Vibrators

Vibration is one massage technique that may be performed better by machine if the vibration is to be done for a long period. Many good mechanical and sound vibration devices are on the market. One for professional use should have varying speeds so that the practitioner can modify the intensity of the application as needed.

Some vibrators are designed to be strapped to the back of the hand as shown in figure 2.31. This allows for the practitioner's hand to touch the recipient as the vibration is applied through the hand. The vibrating hand can be performing other massage techniques such as deep transverse friction at the same time. In this case, the vibration acts as a pain reducer and allows friction to be applied with less pain.

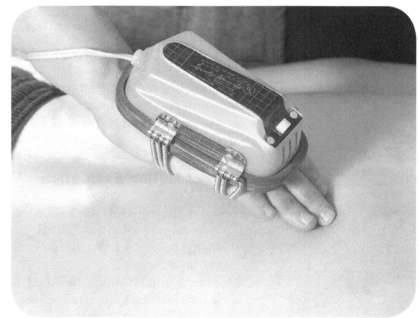

Figure 2.31 Vibration device strapped to the back of the hand.

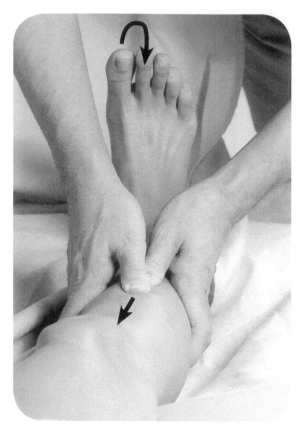

Figure 2.32   Thumb slides during active movement.

Application of Techniques With Active Movement

Massage techniques can be combined with active movement to enhance their overall effects. The athlete moves as instructed while the practitioner applies the massage technique. The combination works well with digital pressure, thumb slides, and broadening techniques.

For example, a broadening technique applied to the quadriceps may be combined with the athlete extending her lower leg at the same time. This particular example is usually performed with the athlete sitting on the side of the massage table. Because muscles broaden when they contract, broadening the tissue manually during contraction magnifies the broadening effect

In another example, active movement of the ankle (i.e., flexion and extension) can be performed while applying thumb slides to the tibialis anterior and retinaculum around the ankle as shown in figure 2.32. The combined effect increases relaxation of the tibialis anterior and helps free up movement of the tendons through the retinaculum. This last technique is appreciated by gymnasts and other athletes whose ankles endure sudden compressive force repeatedly during the practice of their sport.

The movements of the practitioner and the athlete are synchronized as the technique is applied. The practitioner should give the athlete instructions about how the active movement should be performed. This can be accomplished by demonstration or by passive movement of the body part.

BASIC JOINT MOVEMENT TECHNIQUES

Basic joint movement techniques in sports massage include range of motion evaluation, passive joint-mobilizing techniques, and stretches. Thrusting movements to realign joints and "cracking" joints deliberately are *not* in the scope of sports massage.

Range of Motion Evaluation

Range of motion (ROM) refers here to the active or passive movement of a joint for purposes of evaluation. ROM is performed by the athlete himself (active movement) or by the practitioner (passive movement) moving the joint through its functional range.

Moving a joint through its ROM can help the practitioner identify areas of muscle tension that cause shortening, and of adhering myofascial tissues or trigger points that restrict movement. Massage and joint movement techniques are then applied to restore movement to its normal range.

ROM evaluation can serve as a pre- and posttest for the judging progress in improving flexibility in an area. Demonstrated results help the athlete maintain a positive attitude.

ROM can also serve as an evaluation tool to determine whether an injury is structural (i.e., involving the joint itself) or functional (i.e., involving the muscles that move the joint). If the injury is structural, the athlete will feel pain with active and passive movement. If the injury is functional only, the athlete will feel pain with active movement but little pain with passive movement.

Sport professionals working with minor muscular complaints must be able to assess when an athlete should be referred for medical diagnosis. For example, an injury that an athlete self-assesses as a "muscle pull" may actually involve injury to the joint itself. Passive ROM can be used to locate possible structural problems that should be referred immediately to an orthopedic doctor for diagnosis.

Joint-Mobilizing Techniques

Joint-mobilizing techniques involve the passive movement of joints well within their normal range. The practitioner moves the joint in a free, loose, rhythmic manner. Movements can be fast or slow, vigorous or gentle, broad or subtle depending on the therapeutic effects desired.

An example of joint mobilizing is rocking the leg to create movement at the hip. The athlete lies supine with a bolster under the knee. The practitioner places one hand on the top of the thigh and the other hand on the lower leg, and then gently rocks the leg back and forth. This creates inward and outward rotation at the hip. Variations of rocking are rocking compression (see figure 2.17) and *jostling* (see figure 3.3).

Another example of joint mobilization is *wagging* the arm to create movement at the shoulder, elbow, and wrist. The athlete lies supine, and the practitioner grasps the athlete's hand. The athlete's elbow is bent. The practitioner then lifts the arm off the table so that it can swing freely and wags it back and forth (see figure 3.5).

Smaller joints also benefit from mobilizing techniques. All of the joints of the foot can be mobilized using techniques such as scissoring between metatarsals, figure eights of the toes, and wagging the foot with the heels of the hands.

Joint-mobilizing techniques warm up muscles and joints prior to vigorous activity. They can be used to prepare joints and the surrounding muscles for stretching. Gentle, loose passive joint movements also provide feedback to athletes who are unconsciously holding tension in their muscles, signaling them to let go so the free movement can take place.

Passive joint mobilizing is beneficial in the treatment of minor athletic injuries. The gentle passive movement of joints keeps them mobile during tissue healing and helps speed recovery. It can also help reduce muscle tension and voluntary splinting related to pain. Mobilizing joints during injury healing should be pain free and within the athlete's comfort zone.

Stretching

Stretching techniques help increase flexibility, allowing athletes to move freely and easily through their natural range of motion without restrictions or discomfort. Alter (1996) identifies five primary factors that limit flexibility: lack of elasticity of connective tissues in muscles or joints, muscle tension, pain, bone and joint structure limitations, and in the case of active movement, lack of coordination and strength. Stretching, in the context of sports massage, addresses the first three of these factors.

Stretching techniques involve taking a joint to the limit of its functional range of motion and then applying pressure in the direction of the stretch. The goals of stretching in sports massage are to elongate connective tissue and increase its pliability, reduce muscle tension (i.e., chronic contraction), and reeducate the nervous system to allow greater range of motion at a joint. To the extent that massage reduces muscle soreness and pain, it also contributes to an athlete's ease of movement.

Stretching techniques are based on a knowledge of muscle and connective tissue anatomy, as well as neurological processes involving the muscle spindles, Golgi tendon organs, and mechanoreceptors in joints. The following descriptions of stretching techniques include some information about the mechanisms involved in stretching; however, for more detailed scientific explanations, consult sport texts such as *Science of Flexibility* (Alter, 1996).

Types of Stretching

Stretching techniques are classified according to the roles that the athlete and the practitioner have in applying the stretch. The major types of stretching variations are passive, passive-active, active-assisted, active, active-resisted, and passive-resisted.

In *passive* stretches, the athlete is passive while the practitioner applies the technique. In *passive-active* stretching, the practitioner takes a joint to the limit of its range, and then the athlete attempts to hold the position for several seconds. This helps strengthen a weak agonist muscle opposing a tight one. In *active-assisted* stretching, the athlete brings the body part to its limit of range of motion, and then the practitioner increases the stretch by applying pressure in the direction of the stretch. This strengthens a weak agonist opposing a tight muscle and helps establish a pattern for coordinated motion. In *active* stretching, the athlete performs the stretch without assistance using her own muscles.

In *passive-resisted* stretching, resistance is applied to enhance the stretch as in the contract–relax–stretch and contract–relax–stretch using reciprocal inhibition described later. The types of stretching are summarized in table 2.2.

Stretching has a long history in sport conditioning, and different philosophies of stretching have come and gone over the years. It is not within the scope of this text to discuss every stretching theory currently circulating. However, some of the more basic and widely accepted stretching methods used in sports massage are described here.

Because this text focuses primarily on massage techniques, stretches for individual muscles will be presented only as examples of broad categories of stretching techniques. For more detailed instructions on stretches for specific muscles, consult a good stretching text or video.

Table 2.2   Classifications of Stretching

According to the roles of the athlete and the practitioner	
Type	**Description**
Passive	The practitioner applies the stretch; the athlete relaxes.
Passive-active	The practitioner applies the stretch; the athlete holds the position.
Active-assisted	The athlete begins the movement; the practitioner finishes it.
Active	The athlete performs the stretch without aid.
Passive-resisted	The practitioner applies the stretch; the athlete resists the movement at a point in the stretch.
According to the method of application	
Type	**Description**
Ballistic	Bouncing, forceful repeated movements to the limit of motion
Static	Holding the stretch at the limit of motion, slow
Contract–relax–stretch	Contraction of targeted muscle followed by stretch
Contract–relax–stretch with reciprocal inhibition	Contraction of antagonist to the targeted muscle followed by stretch

Ballistic Stretching

The ballistic or bouncing stretch once favored by athletes is now thought to be less effective than other methods and to increase the chance of injury. Ballistic movements activate the protective contraction of the muscles involved (i.e., the stretch reflex) and thus work against lengthening. Forcing the stretch of tissues with sudden movement can also result in tears.

Static Stretching

Static stretching involves placing the body in a position so that the targeted joint is at the limit of its range, and then holding it there for 10 to 30 seconds. The muscles and connective tissue affected typically respond by "letting go" and lengthening, and the stretch can be gently increased. This process can be repeated two or three times. At the finish, the stretch should be released very slowly.

The increase in range of motion that occurs during a static stretch is due to a number of factors. The connective tissue becomes more pliable as a result of warming and the tension applied to the tissues during the stretch. The affected muscles may also have been in partial contraction and then relax and lengthen with the stretch. In addition, when a muscle is stretched, an initial protective rise in tension proportional to the velocity of the stretch occurs. Holding the static stretch beyond this initial phasic component leads to a tonic phase in which the resistance is less and is proportional to the amount of stretch (Alter, 1996).

An example is a passive static stretch of the quadriceps muscles with the athlete in the prone position. In a *passive static stretch*, the athlete relaxes and lets

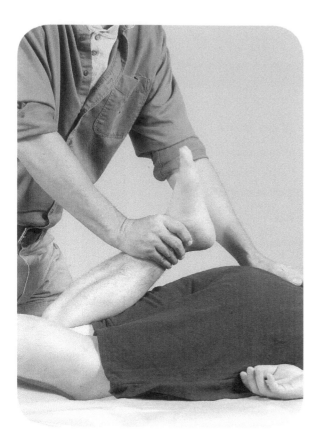

Figure 2.33 Stretch of the quadriceps with athlete prone.

the practitioner perform the movements. The practitioner holds the athlete's leg near the ankle and bends it at the knee so that the heel of the foot moves toward the buttocks muscles (see figure 2.33). As the limit of the range of motion is approached, the practitioner will feel resistance from the quadriceps muscles that are being stretched. Using his own palpation skills and feedback from the athlete, the practitioner determines the limit of the functional range of motion at that time and holds the position. The practitioner feels for a "letting go" or release in the tissues being stretched, and then increases the stretch gently and slowly to the new limit. After repeating this process two or three times, the leg is slowly extended and allowed to rest.

Contract–Relax–Stretch

The *contract–relax–stretch* technique is a form of passive-resisted stretch. In this technique, the athlete contracts the targeted muscle against a resistance supplied by the practitioner for 10 to 15 seconds (i.e., isotonic maximal contraction), and then consciously relaxes the muscle. The practitioner applies the stretch immediately following the relaxation.

To enhance the stretch, the practitioner can ask the athlete to take a deep breath in and then breathe out slowly. The practitioner then applies the stretch on the out-breath.

As an example, we will expand on the quadriceps stretch described in the static stretch section. The practitioner positions the athlete's lower leg near the limit of the stretch. The practitioner then faces the leg so that he can resist the athlete's attempt to extend the leg. The athlete then tries to straighten the leg against the practitioner's resistance using the quadriceps. After about 10 to 15 seconds, the athlete relaxes and takes a deep breath in and then out. The practitioner pushes the lower leg in the direction of the stretch, feeling for the newly established limit.

Contract–Relax–Stretch Using Reciprocal Inhibition

Reciprocal inhibition (RI) is a neuromuscular mechanism that causes an opposing muscle (antagonist) to relax when an active (agonist) muscle contracts. This ensures that the active muscle does not meet resistance from its opposing muscle during performance of an action such as a sport skill. Because the RI mechanism causes muscle relaxation, it can be used to enhance a stretch involving a tense muscle.

Contract–relax–stretch using reciprocal inhibition is another form of passive-resisted stretch. Before applying the stretch in this technique, the athlete contracts the opposing muscles (antagonists) against a resistance supplied by the practitioner. This contraction causes the targeted muscles to relax further and elongate to a greater degree when the stretch is applied.

We will continue the example of the quadriceps stretch, this time using reciprocal inhibition. The practitioner positions the athlete as in the contract–relax–stretch and gets into a position to offer resistance while the athlete tries to flex his leg at the knee. This engages the hamstring muscles (i.e., muscles that oppose the quadriceps). The athlete holds this isometric contraction for 10 to 15 seconds and then relaxes all muscles in the leg.

The RI mechanism will cause the quadriceps to release tension or any partial contraction that may have been present. Thus, when the stretch is applied to the quadriceps, the muscle will elongate further.

SPECIALIZED MASSAGE TECHNIQUES

In addition to the traditional Western massage and joint movements, specialized techniques are integrated into sports massage to address specific tissues and body systems. The four techniques useful in sports massage that are described in this section are positional release, trigger point therapy, myofascial massage, and lymphatic drainage massage. The effects of these specialized techniques are summarized in table 2.3.

Table 2.3 **Specialized Techniques Used in Sports Massage**

Technique	Tissue or system	Uses in sports massage	Description
Positional release	Muscles	Relax tense muscles; relieve spasm	Hold tender points; adjust position
Trigger point therapy	Muscles/tendons	Deactivate trigger points	Ischemic compression, deep thumb slides
Myofascial massage	Fascial tissues	Remove restrictions; increase mobility	Gentle horizontal stretch of soft tissues; skin lifting
Lymphatic drainage massage	Lymph system	Reduce edema; enhance recovery	Gentle movements of skin that open flaps in lymphatic capillary wall

Positional Release

Positional release, also known as strain–counterstrain, was developed by a chiropractor named Lawrence Jones in the early 20th century. It addresses the muscular system and is an effective noninvasive method to ease acute muscle tension or spasm.

Positional release is a simple technique that includes four steps (Chaitow, 1988):

1. Find the tender point in a muscle.
2. Hold the tender point while moving the related joint to a position in which pain is diminished.
3. Hold the position for 90 seconds.
4. Return the area to its neutral resting position.

Tender points are found by palpation of the tissues on or around a tense muscle. A tender point is a specific sore spot that elicits pain when pressed. This point is used to find the correct position for helping the tense muscle to relax.

The positional release of a tight latissimus dorsi muscle is demonstrated in figure 2.34, a through d. The tender spot must be pressed with enough pressure to monitor its tenderness, but not so much pressure as to cause tissue damage.

Positional release is an effective technique that does not involve the more intense discomfort associated with some deep-muscle techniques. Positional release can be used to address chronic muscle tension as well as acute situations.

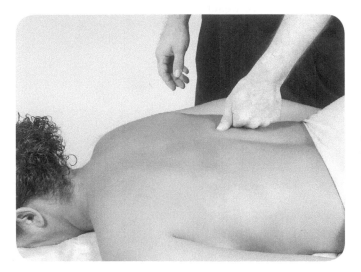

Figure 2.34a Positional release step 1: Find and hold the tender point.

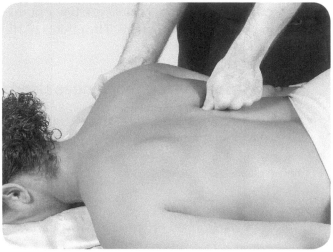

Figure 2.34b Positional release step 2: Move the associated joint to a position of diminished pain.

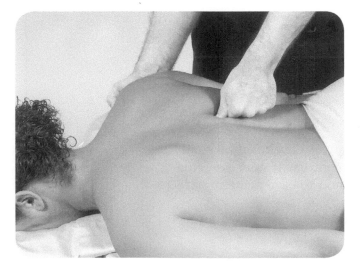

Figure 2.34c Positional release step 3: Hold the tender point in the position of diminished pain for 90 seconds.

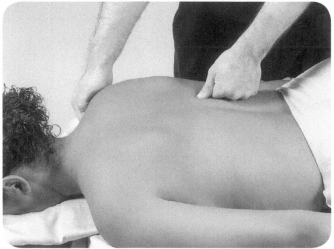

Figure 2.34d Positional release step 4: Return the area to its neutral resting position.

Trigger Point Therapy

Trigger point therapy, also known as neuromuscular therapy, was pioneered by Janet Travell, MD, in the 1960s. It involves deactivation of trigger points (TrPs) in muscle and related connective tissues.

Trigger points (TrPs) undoubtedly account for much of the muscle pain and dysfunction experienced by athletes in training. TrPs are caused by acute muscle overload, repetitive strain, overwork, fatigue, poor posture or body mechanics, blunt trauma, and chilling. They typically occur in muscles and tendons used most often in a particular sport.

TrPs are palpated as taut bands of tissue that elicit exquisite pain when pressed and refer pain if active. Travell and Simons (1983) defined a trigger point as follows:

> . . . a focus of hyperirritability in a tissue that, when compressed, is locally tender and, if sufficiently hypersensitive, gives rise to referred pain and tenderness, and sometimes to referred autonomic phenomena and distortion of proprioception. (p. 4)

Signs of TrPs include dull, aching, or deep referred pain; variable irritability over time; stiffness and weakness in the involved muscle; restricted range of motion; pain on contraction; and pain on stretching. The pain experienced will often be out of proportion to the pressure applied directly to the area and may be felt either in the immediate area or in a remote place on the body.

Ischemic compression is a technique used to deactivate trigger points. It involves the application of direct digital pressure with enough force to cause blanching in the tissues. Ischemic compression is held for 15 to 45 seconds while the practitioner feels for a release or softening of the trigger point, or diminishing of the local or referred pain. The technique is repeated two to four times.

The application of ischemic compression should be preceded by the warming of tissues with massage. Techniques that can be combined with ischemic compression in deactivating trigger points include deep sliding movements with the thumb over the taut band of tissue, kneading, broadening, and fine vibration. Positional release may also be used for TrPs. Circulatory massage techniques such as sliding and kneading can be applied to move out metabolic wastes once the trigger point is relieved. Stretching techniques should be applied after massage to reeducate the muscle to its increased length after deactivation of the TrP. Figure 2.35, a and b, shows the application of ischemic compression to a trigger point on the pectoralis minor, followed by a stretch of the muscle.

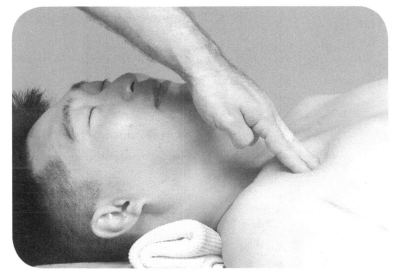

Figure 2.35a   Ischemic compression to a trigger point in the pectoralis minor.

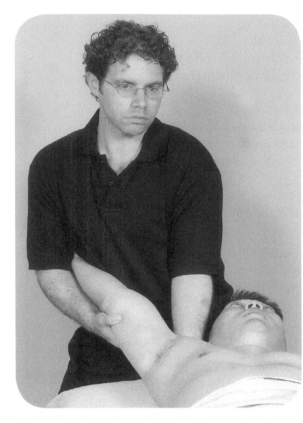

Figure 2.35b Stretching the pectoralis minor after trigger point release.

Trigger point charts pinpoint common TrP locations and identify their zones of reference. These charts are useful for locating TrPs using athlete feedback about the pain they are experiencing. Travell and Simons (1983, 1992, 1999) have written the bible on trigger points for the major muscles of the body.

Myofascial Massage

Myofascial massage, also called myofascial release, grew out of the work of Ida Rolf in the 1970s. Myofascial massage involves restoring mobility and removing restrictions in fascial tissues using soft tissue stretching techniques.

Fascial tissues of particular interest in sports massage include subcutaneous fascia, fascia related to the musculature, and fascial sheaths such as retinaculae (i.e., bands or straps) at the ankle and wrist. Unrestricted myofascial tissues enhance ease of movement and improve sport performance.

The goals of myofascial techniques are to make fascial tissues more pliable and to break cross-links or adhesions. This is done by stretching tissues and applying a shearing force horizontally that separates tissues that have become "stuck" together.

Guidelines for myofascial massage outlined in Benjamin and Tappan (2005) include the following:

1. Use observation, palpation skills, and knowledge of myofascial anatomy to identify areas of fascial restriction.
2. Choose techniques suitable for the area and depth at which you are working.
3. Use little or no lubricant so that you can feel restrictions and avoid sliding.
4. Make gentle contact and enter tissues slowly until a point of resistance is felt.
5. Shift tissues horizontally once you are at the correct depth.
6. Hold the stretch of tissues until they release, usually in two to five minutes.
7. Release will feel like a "melting" or "letting go."
8. Flow with the tissues.
9. Exit the tissues slowly and with awareness.
10. Let fascial tissues rest and integrate change after the stretch.

Myofascial massage techniques include skin lifting and rolling described previously, which address subcutaneous fascia. The multiple-digit overlay hand position and the forearm are used to apply a horizontal stretch to deeper soft tissues. Other techniques such as the cross-handed stretch to the back have been developed to achieve myofascial goals (see Manheim, 2001).

The study of myofascial anatomy facilitates the effective application of myofascial techniques (see also Schultz & Feitis, 1996).

Lymphatic Drainage Massage

Lymphatic drainage massage (LDM), also called manual lymph drainage, was advanced by Emil and Estid Vodder in the 1930s. LDM uses gentle soft tissue techniques to move interstitial fluid into the lymph capillaries, and lymph fluid through the lymphatic vessels and nodes.

The uses of LDM techniques in sports massage include local applications to reduce edema around joints, to increase circulation during injury rehabilitation, and to enhance healing after surgery. General applications of LDM aid in recovery from strenuous activity and can benefit athletes with allergies and those recovering from the common cold or seasonal viruses.

General circulatory massage emphasizes sliding and kneading techniques that enhance the overall circulation of blood and lymph in the larger vessels. LDM techniques specifically focus on the 70 percent of the lymphatic vessels (i.e., capillaries) located in the skin.

LDM techniques use very light pressure, just enough to move the skin. The gentle stretching of the skin in the direction of the targeted lymph node opens the overflaps between cells in the walls of the lymph capillaries. Tiny filaments attach the overflaps to the skin tissues, and so movement of the skin opens the flaps. This allows interstitial fluid to enter the tiny vessels. If too much pressure is used, the flaps close and the fluid cannot enter the capillaries.

Techniques are repeated in the same spot six to eight times. They are performed in sequence following the drainage pattern of the lymph system (see Kelly, 2002). LDM techniques developed by the Vodders include stationary circles and the scoop, pump, and rotary techniques.

PALPATION

Perhaps the most basic and crucial skill in giving sports massage is palpation. At its simplest level, *palpation* is the ability to locate with the hands specific structures such as bony landmarks, individual muscles and tendons, and their attachments. This ability adds the quality of specificity to the session. For example, figure 3.9 shows palpation and friction to the attachments of extensor muscles near the elbow. (See also Biel, 2001.)

During passive joint-mobilizing techniques and stretching, information about the condition of a joint can be surmised through certain qualities of the movements (e.g., crepitations, drag, or end feel). Palpatory information also helps locate the source of resistance in range of motion evaluation.

In addition, massage specialists learn to recognize the texture of the soft tissues, their degree of pliability, and the difference between good muscle tone and a tense muscle. For example, hypertonic muscle is hard and ropelike, whereas healthy muscle tissue is firm yet elastic. Massage specialists can also feel where tissues are adhering and identify conditions such as scarring, fibrosis, and edema. They can locate the taut bands of trigger points and feel subtle resistance in fascial stretches.

More important, massage specialists can learn to detect changes in the tissues and qualities of movement during a session in response to techniques, or from one session to the next. This provides important feedback about the effectiveness of applications.

In this chapter the basic techniques of sports massage have been described including hand positions, Western massage techniques, specialized techniques, and palpation skills. These basic techniques are used separately, but more often in combination to achieve specific goals related to the athlete's health and to sport performance. Variations of these techniques are endless, and massage specialists continually create new versions as they gain further training and experience.

Chapter 3 describes in more detail how to apply these basic techniques as restorative massage. The three major aspects of restoration are recovery, remedial applications, and rehabilitation.

STUDY QUESTIONS

1. How are the hands and fingers positioned to apply massage techniques?
2. What are the eight basic sports massage techniques and their effects?
3. How are joint movements used in sports massage? Identify three applications.
4. How are passive-assisted stretches used to increase flexibility? Give examples.
5. For what purpose is positional release used in sports massage? How is it performed?
6. What is a trigger point, and how are TrPs deactivated using manual techniques?
7. How are fascial restrictions released using manual techniques? Of what benefit is this to athletes?
8. How do lymphatic drainage massage techniques enhance lymph flow? When are they used in sports massage?
9. Which palpation skills are useful in sports massage? How do massage specialists use the information they get from palpation?

RESTORATIVE SPORTS MASSAGE

LEARNING OUTCOMES

1. Describe the three major applications of restorative massage.
2. Explain the guidelines for recovery massage.
3. Distinguish between remedial and rehabilitation sports massage applications.
4. Give examples of remedial and rehabilitation applications for common sports injuries.

RESTORATIVE MASSAGE AND ITS APPLICATIONS

Sports are physically, mentally, and emotionally demanding for athletes of all ages and skill levels. Players are always at risk of injury, and the training required for top performance stresses the body and mind. Practice and competition can leave athletes tired, drained of energy, and psychologically depleted.

Helping athletes recover from bouts of activity and restoring athletes to pre-injury levels of physical and psychological fitness are the goals of restorative massage. Taken a step further, restorative massage can help athletes exceed their previous levels of fitness to avoid future injury.

Restorative massage has three major applications: recovery, remedial, and rehabilitation. These categories represent a range of severity of the athlete's condition or injury, from simple stress resulting from strenuous activity, to minor injuries, to conditions that disable the athlete.

○ *Recovery* massage applications are for the uninjured athlete recovering from a strenuous workout or competition.

○ *Remedial* massage applications are for athletes with minor to moderate injuries.

○ *Rehabilitation* massage applications are part of a comprehensive treatment plan for athletes with severe injuries or following surgery.

This chapter explains how massage is used to help restore athletes to optimal condition from various degrees of debility or disability. Examples of massage applications for treating several common sports injuries are presented.

RECOVERY MASSAGE

Sports massage given after a strenuous workout or competition can enhance the athlete's physical, mental, and emotional recovery from the stress of the activity. It augments the body's own healing process and helps the athlete maintain a state of dynamic equilibrium. Sports massage facilitates recovery by increasing circulation (which promotes better cell nutrition and removal of waste products), relaxing tight muscles, and inducing general body–mind relaxation.

The duration of a recovery massage session depends on its proximity in time to the strenuous event. Soon after an event or hard workout, the session should be shorter, usually about 30 minutes. Several hours later, or the following day, a recovery session may last an hour.

Techniques used for recovery include deep sliding, compression, kneading, skin rolling, circular friction, positional release, joint mobilizing, and stretching. The tempo is relaxing, and the application is to the entire body with specific attention to the muscle groups most stressed during the activity. Deep breathing and other relaxation techniques are valuable adjuncts to massage for recovery. Time spent in a whirlpool, sauna, steam room, or hot shower before the massage can prepare the athlete for deeper relaxation.

General guidelines for recovery sports massage are as follows:

○ Aim to improve circulation and promote muscular and general relaxation.

- ○ Include techniques such as sliding, compression, kneading, skin rolling, circular friction, positional release, joint mobilizing, and stretching.
- ○ Spend more time on areas stressed in the activity.
- ○ Vary the duration from 30 to 60 minutes depending on the proximity in time to the activity.
- ○ Suggest a hot shower, whirlpool, sauna, or steam room before the massage.
- ○ Include deep breathing and other relaxation methods.

Athletes and their coaches want quick recovery and restoration to normalcy, especially during the competitive season. Although the sports massage specialist is the ideal candidate for giving recovery massage, it is a relatively simple application and can be learned by coaches, athletic trainers, teammates, and even family members.

Recovery Massage Without Oil

Recovery sports massage can be given without using oil or other lubricant (see King, 1993). The athlete may wear shorts and a T-shirt or a warm-up suit for modesty and warmth. Massage techniques that can be applied over clothing include compression, kneading, circular friction, broadening, skin rolling, positional release, rocking, jostling, and stretching. For each body region, warm the

---

HISTORY BRIEF 4

Massage at the YMCA

In 1915 when R. Tait McKenzie described the YMCA's program of exercise, the rubdown was already an established part of the routine. According to McKenzie, workouts at the YMCA included a mixture of Swedish and German gymnastics and games, "ending with a bath and a rub down" (p. 170).

The Dayton Association in Ohio established a School of Health Services and Massage in 1937 to train massage practitioners. A Health Service Operators Society was formed in 1942 to advance health services at the YMCA and to "combat the abuses of commercial bath houses and the unethical conduct of 'cure-all' agents in the health field" (Williams, 1943, p. 30). The society was active through the 1950s.

By 1943, a total of 274 YMCAs in the United States operated health service sections that offered massage. "The technician uses massage, baths (shower, steam, electricity cabinet), ultraviolet radiation (artificial and natural sunlight), infrared (heat), instruction in relaxation and in some cases directed exercise. The adult members secure a relief from tensions, gain a sense of well-being, give attention to personal fitness and develop habits designed to build and maintain optimum health and physical efficiency throughout the lifespan" (Frierwood, 1953, p. 21).

tissues first, follow with more specific work, and end with nonspecific connecting and finishing techniques.

Prone Position

The athlete lies facedown on the massage table. Place a bolster or rolled towel under the ankles for support, or let the feet hang off the end of the table.

Legs

Begin warming up the entire left leg and hip using rocking compression and jostling. Follow with compression, kneading, and broadening techniques on the large muscles of the leg starting with the buttocks, then upper leg, lower leg, and finishing with the feet.

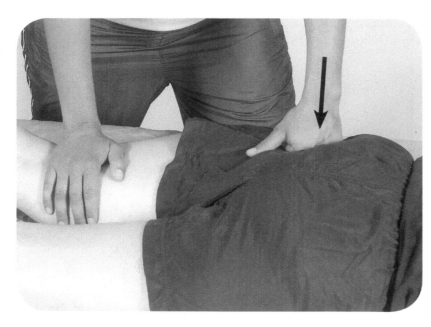

Compression and kneading are effective on the large buttocks muscles. Figure 3.1 shows compression on the buttocks using the fist. Use broadening, kneading, and jostling on the upper leg, and then repeat on the lower leg. For a gentle stretch of the quadriceps, bend the leg at the knee, bringing the heel of the foot toward the buttocks. Use the passive-resisted techniques described in chapter 2 to enhance the stretch. With the lower leg flexed at a 90-degree angle, perform some joint-mobilizing techniques for the ankle. Then hold the foot off the table with one hand and apply compressions to the bottom of the foot with your other hand.

Finish with some light palmar sliding strokes or light percussion over the clothing from the foot to the buttocks to reconnect the leg kinesthetically and create a feeling of wholeness. Repeat the entire leg sequence on the right side.

Figure 3.1 Compression on the buttocks using a fist.

Back

Use compression and rocking compression to warm up the muscles of the back. Follow with kneading the shoulders. Use circular friction along the paraspinal muscles as shown in figure 3.2. Perform skin rolling to the entire back, especially along the spine and over the scapulae. Finish with light sliding movements or light percussion over the back from the shoulders to the hips.

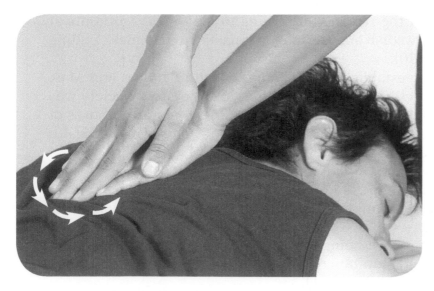

Figure 3.2 Circular friction on the erector spinae muscles.

Supine Position

The athlete lies faceup on the massage table. Place a bolster under the knees to take pressure off the lower back. A small towel may be used as a neck roll for support.

Legs

Warm up the front of the left leg using compression and rocking compression. Begin specific work on the upper leg applying broadening, kneading, and jostling techniques. Add circular friction around the knees. Apply compression along the tibialis anterior, pressing away from the tibia. Use circular friction around the ankle. Apply thumb slides to the dorsal foot and mobilize the foot bones. Finish with light palmar sliding movements from ankle to hip, and then jostle the muscles of the leg while moving your hands from the hip to the foot (see figure 3.3). Repeat on the right side.

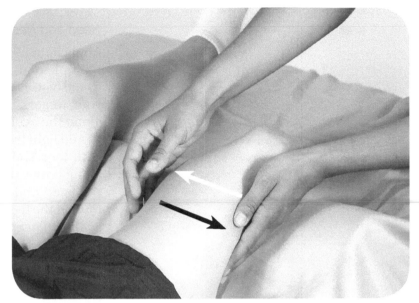

Figure 3.3   Jostling the leg from side to side.

Chest

Use light compression with the fist to warm the pectoral muscles. Follow with circular friction with the fingertips along the attachments on the sternum. Stretch the arms overhead. Finish with light tapping over the chest. Avoid touching breast tissue in women.

Arm and Shoulder

Gently squeeze the arm in your two hands, moving from the armpit to the wrist (see figure 3.4). Repeat twice to warm the area. Continue with more specific massage in sequence from the upper arm to the lower arm, wrist, and hand.

Perform compressions, kneading, and broadening on the shoulder and upper arm. Use the same techniques on the lower arm, varying your hand position to accommodate the smaller size.

Use circular friction with the thumbs around the wrist. Mobilize all of the joints of the hand. Perform thumb slides on the palm of the hand.

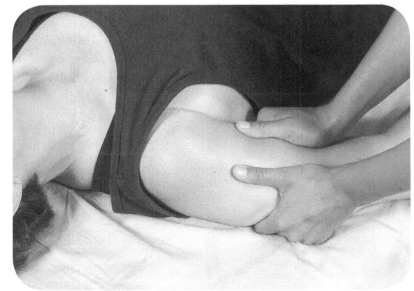

Figure 3.4   Squeezing and broadening the muscles of the arm using two hands.

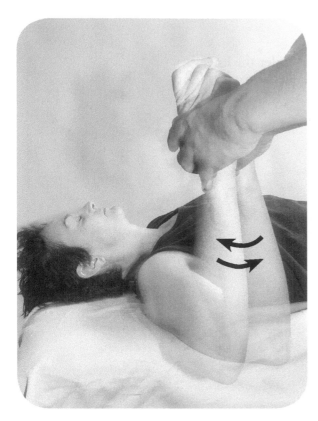

Figure 3.5 Mobilizing the arm and shoulder using a wagging movement.

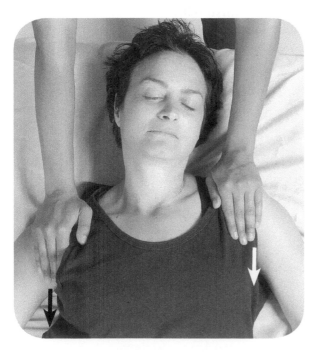

Figure 3.6 Mobilizing the shoulders using alternating pressing toward the feet.

To mobilize and relax the entire arm, grasp the hand and bend the arm to a 90-degree angle, lift the arm slightly off of the table, and then wag the arm back and forth creating movement at the shoulder, elbow, and wrist (see figure 3.5). Finish with light sliding movements from the shoulder to the hand.

Head and Neck

Apply light friction to the back and sides of the neck using multiple-digit placement. The joints of the neck will mobilize as you push up on the neck muscles with the tips of your fingers. Apply digital compression to the muscles along the occipital ridge.

Add light friction to the sides and top of the head. Finish with long sliding strokes from the shoulder to the head along both sides of the body. To end the session, stand at the head and mobilize the shoulders by pressing them toward the feet with a catlike movement, alternating sides as shown in figure 3.6. Hold the shoulders lightly for a few seconds before breaking contact.

REMEDIAL APPLICATIONS

Injuries and debilitating conditions occur with unfortunate regularity in both amateur and professional sports. Even minor problems can hamper athletic performance and can lead to more serious injury if left unchecked. Massage therapy intended to treat these minor conditions is called remedial massage.

The general intent of remedial massage is to restore the athlete's optimal level of physical, mental, and emotional fitness, and perhaps even exceed his previous level to prevent further problems. Remedial massage applications are specific in their approach and are results oriented.

The primary objective of remedial sports massage is to reduce or eliminate the complaint, which is typically pain and dysfunction. After pain and other symptoms have been addressed, methods to prevent recurrence of the complaint are investigated. This includes investigation of the biomechanical factors that caused or that resulted from the initial complaint. A comprehensive approach will minimize the potential of future injury.

Because the public has direct access to sports massage specialists, athletes with minor problems often seek out sports massage practitioners as the first source for consultation. The massage professional has the responsibility of knowing what can be treated safely and what should be referred to a primary care provider for diagnosis prior to massage. Continuing education in remedial applications of sports massage is recommended before treating even minor athletic injuries.

A remedial sports massage session may last from 5 to 15 minutes with treatment applied specifically at the injury site. However, an entire session may extend to 30 minutes to include warming the tissues and other preparation. The tempo of technique application varies with the specific goals of the session, but should be slow enough for the exactness and care required when working with injured tissues. Remedial treatments are usually given two to three times a week depending on the timing of the tissue repair process. The frequency of visits decreases as the athlete returns to normal activity.

Remedial sports massage is usually part of a total treatment plan that includes rest or activity modification, application of heat or ice, and simple home exercises and stretching. Education about the causes for the onset of the condition and how to avoid them in the future is also important. As part of the athlete's health team, the sports massage specialist is in a good position to reinforce instructions given to the athlete by the athletic trainer, physical therapist, or physician. The massage specialist may also advise athletes about adjunct modalities in cases of minor or subclinical complaints.

REHABILITATION APPLICATIONS

Rehabilitation massage applications are applied in the context of an overall treatment plan for a specific diagnosed injury or conditions that disable an athlete and require the care of a physician. Remedial applications cross into the category of rehabilitation if the condition is severe enough to send the athlete to a health care provider for treatment, and she discontinues her sport while she heals. Massage then becomes part of an overall rehabilitation plan that involves other modalities and possibly prescribed medication.

Rehabilitation is often the job of a health care team, rather than one person. The massage practitioner assisting in the rehabilitation of an athlete works closely with the physician, athletic trainer, or physical therapist on the case.

The applications of massage for rehabilitation aim toward reducing pain, edema, and spasm; increasing the circulation of blood and lymph; forming healthy scar tissue and breaking adhesions; promoting early mobility; reducing muscle tension; and reducing general anxiety and stress. However, there are no easy formulas for the use of massage with severe injuries because each athlete and injury presents its own unique situation. (See Bahr & Maehlum, 2004; Cash, 1996; Landry & Bernhardt, 2003.)

Twelve examples of remedial and rehabilitation sports massage applications are described in this section. They range from relatively minor problems such as loss of flexibility and muscle tension and postexercise soreness and edema; to moderately serious conditions such as subclinical tendinitis, low-grade strains and sprains, and emotional stress; to more serious conditions such as tennis elbow, shin splints, plantar fasciitis, and recovery from surgery. The examples of massage applications are not protocols or formulas but descriptions of how massage might be applied in a specific case.

1. Loss of Flexibility and Muscle Tension

Muscle tension and abnormalities in connective tissues cause loss of flexibility. The factors associated with limited range of motion that can be addressed with sports massage include the following:

- Muscle–tendon shortening from inactivity
- Chronic muscle tension from overactivity
- Voluntary or involuntary splinting from pain in muscles and joints
- Thickening of fascia in and around a muscle or muscle group
- Fascial adhesions
- Excessive scar tissue or scar tissue in a place that limits movement
- Edema or excessive fluid around a joint
- Emotional stress and anxiety
- Excessive stimulation (e.g., being too hyped-up)

When developing a session strategy, determining the main causes of loss of flexibility is important. Although muscle tension is often the chief suspect, further examination is required. For example, a joint with a structural problem from a past injury or arthritis may exhibit restricted ROM while the surrounding musculature is flexible and relaxed. Conversely, an athlete may be hypermobile at a joint yet have tension in surrounding musculature. The sports massage specialist uses palpation skills to determine the condition of the musculature and degree of tension present. When muscle tension is the cause of limited ROM, massage can be very effective in improving flexibility.

A distinction exists between chronic and acute muscle tension. The sports massage approach for these two situations is different as described in the following sections.

Chronic Muscle Tension.   Chronic conditions develop slowly. The possible causes of chronic muscle tension include poor posture, repetitive use, inefficient biomechanical patterns, and unconscious holding of tension and emotional stress. The tissues involved will exhibit signs of fascial thickening, trigger points, adhesions, ischemia, and sometimes crepitation. In some cases of chronic tension the complaint is burning neuralgia or myositis; in others there is a dulling of sensation in the area. Athletes typically experience significant pain when pressure is applied. Other symptoms include fatigue and loss of flexibility and power of the muscle involved. These symptoms combine to set up the pain-spasm-pain cycle that perpetuates the condition.

Massage techniques that increase circulation, cause fascial lengthening, reduce adhesions, and deactivate trigger points help relieve chronic muscle tension. These include deep sliding strokes, deep transverse friction, compression, broadening, digital pressure to TrPs, positional release, myofascial massage, jostling, and stretching. Working within the optimal therapy zone provides significant and quick results.

Acute Muscle Tension.   Acute muscle tension can result from a sudden forceful muscle contraction or stretch, blunt trauma directly to the muscle, recent overuse that causes muscle soreness, or emotional tension (e.g., performance anxiety). In these cases deep massage is likely to aggravate the tissues.

Juhan (1987) suggested that force cannot be used to make a muscle relax or lengthen, and that manual techniques should be applied slowly and in a nonthreatening manner to effect relaxation. He maintained that physical and emotional pleasure is essential in "interrupting self-perpetuating cycles of excess tension," and that pain and discomfort are counterproductive because they trigger a protective response (p. 206). This view echoes Galen's advice centuries before that in "rubbing" after exercise the "hard kinds" should be avoided, and that movements should be quick and soft "to carry off the excretions and soften the tense parts" (Johnson, 1866, p. 25). This picture runs counter to the stereotypical big, bruising masseur or masseuse pummeling muscles into submission while the client screams in pain.

Massage techniques that increase circulation, reduce local nerve excitation, evoke a neuromuscular relaxation effect, and produce general relaxation are effective in reducing acute muscle tension. These include sliding strokes, compression, kneading, vibration, jostling, joint mobilizing, and passive and contract–relax stretches that use reciprocal inhibition. Techniques must be applied gently with gradual deepening to prevent further tensing of the muscles involved.

The massage specialist can also suggest ways to reduce the factors that caused the chronic or acute muscle tension, and teach the athlete self-massage and stretching for the most stressed muscles. Coaches can help correct inefficient biomechanical patterns or improper use of equipment. Athletes can also learn relaxation techniques such as progressive relaxation, autonomic suggestion, and deep breathing to reduce stress and tension overall.

2. Postexercise Muscle Soreness

Two types of postexercise muscle soreness are *acute muscle pain* and *delayed-onset soreness*. Acute muscle pain is thought to be related to a condition of *ischemia* (i.e., lack of sufficient blood) brought on by intense exercise of short duration. This type of pain decreases when circulation is increased to the area.

Delayed-onset soreness, however, "increases from 2 to 3 days following strenuous exercise, usually peaks in intensity 24 to 48 hours post exercise, and thereafter slowly diminishes disappearing at 5 to 7 days after exercise" (Yackzan, Adams, & Francis, 1984, p. 159). Five different theories have been proposed to explain delayed-onset muscle soreness: tonic muscle spasm, torn tissue (microtears), connective tissue damage, accumulation of waste products in the tissues, and low-level edema. Any of these conditions, or a combination of factors, can result in various degrees of soreness and stiffness after exercise.

Massage is an effective treatment for both types of muscle soreness because one of its primary effects is increased circulation of blood and lymph fluid. Increased circulation brings cellular nutrients, carries away metabolites, reduces edema, and promotes faster healing of injured tissues.

Effective circulatory massage includes a combination of sliding, pumping and rocking compression, and kneading techniques. The pressure used in applying massage to sore muscles should be light at first and then increase gradually as circulation improves and pain decreases. Joint-mobilizing techniques and stretching can be incorporated to enhance healing of the area.

3. Edema

Edema is the abnormal accumulation of fluid in the interstitial spaces of tissues. This excess fluid causes noticeable and palpable swelling, soreness and pain, and restricted movement around joints. Edema is present in most injuries and may also accompany delayed-onset soreness, minor strains and sprains, inflammation, and tendinitis. Swelling around joints can also result from the stress of strenuous exercise.

The edema typically dealt with in sports massage is associated with an injury or inflammation from activity. This type of edema is relieved with light pressure applied in long sliding strokes. Pressure should be applied broadly using the palm of the hand or the soft surface of several fingers, always moving in a distal-to-proximal direction on the limbs.

Lymphatic drainage massage (LDM) techniques that target the lymph capillaries are also effective for reducing edema. A simple LDM technique can be applied with the soft flat surface of the fingers. Place the fingers on the skin over the edema and gently stretch the skin in the direction of the next proximal lymph node. Pressure is then released and the skin is allowed to snap back. The movement is repeated rhythmically six to eight times in one place before moving to another spot. This repetitive action helps open the lymph capillaries so that fluid in the area can be absorbed more easily into the lymph vessels and carried away.

When an injury is healing well (i.e., pain and inflammation are reduced), but swelling is still present, deep and slow sliding movements applied to the area can help push the accumulated fluids along. Massage is contraindicated in cases of acute inflammation.

4. Subclinical Tendinitis

Tendinitis (i.e., tendon inflammation) is a common condition among athletes that results from a variety of factors such as poor body mechanics, repetitive motion, irritation, or sudden increase in workload. Once tendinitis sets in, it causes pain and interferes with sport performance.

One of the benefits of regular maintenance massage is that the massage practitioner can detect subclinical tendinitis during a massage session. *Subclinical* refers to a condition that does not present overt symptoms. Subclinical tendinitis is painful under the pressure of massage, but the athlete reports being unaware that a problem existed beforehand. A common comment is, "My tendon was fine until you pressed on it!" In reality, the tendon was not "fine," and if left alone would probably develop into a full tendinitis condition with pain and dysfunction.

If subclinical tendinitis is detected during a massage session, the athlete, coach, and athletic trainer can begin a comprehensive treatment plan. Quick action can prevent a more serious problem from developing.

The standard treatment for subclinical and moderate tendinitis includes cryotherapy (e.g., ice massage), nonsteroidal anti-inflammatory drugs (NSAIDs), deep transverse friction massage, modification of activity, and correction of poor biomechanics. The use of ice and NSAIDs is important when the treatment plan also calls for deep transverse friction, which can irritate the tissues. Relaxing and elongating the muscle involved will reduce stress on the tendon and provide a better environment for healing.

In severe cases of tendinitis, deep transverse friction may be contraindicated until the condition has improved. Massage to reduce tension and spasm in the associated muscle is beneficial in this early stage of healing, and deep transverse friction may be added to the treatment once inflammation has subsided.

5. Tenosynovitis

Sheathed tendons are found in the wrists, hands, ankles, and feet. Inflammation of these tendons and/or the surrounding tenosynovial sheath is called tenosynovitis. This condition is typically caused by mechanical irritation of the tendon resulting from repetitive strain or poor biomechanics.

Symptoms of acute tenosynovitis include pain, heat, swelling, and stiffness. There may be a "gritty" feel or sound as the tendon moves through the sheath. Massage is contraindicated in the acute stage of inflammation (Werner, 2002).

Massage therapy for tenosynovitis is similar to that for tendinitis except that the tendon must be stretched taut during the application of deep transverse friction. Cyriax and Cyriax (1993) explained that "the manual rolling of the tendon sheath to and fro against the tendon serves to smooth off the roughened surfaces." (p. 19)

For complete healing, the cause of the irritation must be eliminated. The coach or athletic trainer can help identify and correct any contributing biomechanical factors.

6. Strains

A *strain* is damage to a part of a muscle, fascia, or tendon brought on by overuse (i.e., chronic strain) or by overstress (i.e., acute strain). An acute strain is usually related to sudden changes of tension in a muscle created by something like a violent stretch or rapid contraction. Sudden bursts of power such as charging to the net in tennis, sprinting in track, or landing a dismount with hyperextended knees in gymnastics are some examples of activities that result in strains. A strain may also be caused by decelerating a high-speed movement such as when pitching a baseball.

Grade 1 Strain. A grade 1 strain is characterized by low-grade inflammation, edema, and mild discomfort in use. There may be no apparent loss of range of motion or strength, and there is no palpable defect in the tissues. However, partial tearing or microtears may be present, and spasm or edema may cause pain.

Treatment of a grade 1 strain consists of ice and massage. Begin with light sliding strokes to improve circulation and decrease edema in the area. Next, apply sliding and kneading using moderate pressure and other techniques to reduce muscle tension or spasm. As pain subsides, more vigorous massage and massage to the specific injury site will further promote tissue healing.

For example, massage a mildly strained quadriceps with a combination of sliding, vibration, and kneading. Keep the pressure and pace of the massage lighter and slower at first and then increase pressure and pace as the pain subsides, either within one session or over a series of spaced sessions.

Grade 2 Strain. A grade 2 strain has definite inflammation and edema with possible hemorrhaging (i.e., bruising). The athlete will experience severe discomfort with use, voluntary or involuntary muscle splinting, and discernable loss of ROM and strength in the affected muscle. There will be a palpable lesion in the injured muscle or tendon.

Treatment includes the application of ice, rest, and modification of movement. Massage directly over the injury site is contraindicated. However, massage of the muscles proximal to the injured area may help reduce edema and release muscle tension in the area. Stay well within the athlete's comfort zone when massaging the area.

Several days postinjury, more vigorous massage may be applied around, but not directly on, the injury site to assist in the removal of debris caused by the hemorrhage. Gentle sliding movements, or lymphatic drainage techniques, may be applied directly over the injury site to help reduce edema, staying within the athlete's comfort zone.

Once the area has had significant reduction in swelling and the hemorrhage begins to dissipate, apply moderate massage to the entire length of the injured muscle. More vigorous massage may be added if it doesn't cause the athlete discomfort. During the final stages of healing, apply deep transverse friction directly to the injury site to address adhesions and scarring.

Massage is very effective at speeding recovery from grade 2 strains. However, it must be applied with awareness to avoid further trauma to the injured tissues. If the injury is severe or if you question the appropriateness of treatment at a given time, refer the athlete to a sports medicine physician for diagnosis. Only massage practitioners with specific training in treating musculoskeletal injuries should attempt to treat grade 2 strains with massage.

Grade 3 Strain. Grade 3 strains are characterized by severe inflammation, edema with discoloration, and severely impaired function of the affected muscle. There will be a definite palpable lesion, possibly accompanied by muscle "bunching." Always refer suspected grade 3 strains to a physician for diagnosis. Treatment may include surgical intervention. In the absence of surgery and with referral by a physician, massage may be performed as in a grade 2 strain. Timelines for healing should be extended appropriately, and complete rest of the area should be encouraged.

7. Sprains

Sprains are injuries to ligaments and other stabilizing structures caused by the sudden forced stretch of a joint beyond its normal ROM. Sprains range from those exhibiting no significant loss of function (grade 1) to those with complete rupture and loss of function (grade 3). Sprains can be serious enough to require surgical intervention. In addition, sprains and fractures can have similar symptoms, so it is best to refer most sprains to a physician for diagnosis.

In the early stages of healing of any sprain, use rest, ice, compression, elevation, and stabilization (RICES) as first aid and until symptoms subside. Gentle joint mobilizations that do not cause pain may be applied in the early stages and continued throughout the healing process to help keep joints supple and hasten the return to normal ROM. Sliding strokes may be applied to the surrounding area to improve circulation and reduce edema.

Muscles in the area of a sprain often become tense from the trauma itself and the accompanying pain. In addition, other muscles may become tense from protective holding or from modified movement patterns such as limping with a knee or ankle sprain. This muscle tension can cause added pain and debility. Massage can be applied to reduce tension in the affected musculature.

After the acute phase of a sprain, deep transverse friction applied directly to the injury site can assist in the formation of a functional scar. Figure 3.7 demonstrates deep friction being applied to a lateral ankle ligament.

Deep transverse friction can also prevent and break adhesions. Ligaments and related soft structures are designed to slide over the bones they are supporting. A healing ligament will sometimes adhere to skeletal tissues it comes in contact with. These adhesions can cause chronic pain and a cycle of injury-healing-reinjury as a result of the dysfunctional condition of the joint. Deep transverse friction can eliminate the adhesions and restore the structure to its optimal function.

Strengthening exercises should be performed as part of the healing strategy. Exercises not only restore related muscles to their preinjury condition, but also add dynamic stability to the joint itself and help compensate for loss of static stability resulting from postsprain ligament weakness.

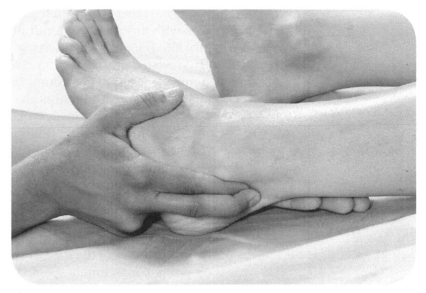

Figure 3.7 Deep transverse friction applied to a lateral ankle ligament.

8. Emotional Stress

Moderate stress can be stimulating and invigorating. However, the pressures of training and competition added to stresses from school, work, family, friends, and other life situations can result in nearly debilitating levels of stress (i.e., distress). Massage can help relieve stress, especially when used in conjunction with other stress reduction measures such as deep breathing, meditation, progressive relaxation, proper nutrition, and lifestyle habits such as adequate sleep and recreation. Some cases of emotional stress are best referred to psychotherapists.

Massage used for stress reduction includes techniques and qualities of application that evoke the physiological relaxation response described in chapter 2. Apply massage for general relaxation and for specific tight areas. The most effective techniques for deep relaxation are combinations of long sliding strokes and kneading. Techniques that tend to stimulate, such as percussion and friction, should be avoided. The quality of the massage should be smooth and flowing, at a slow to moderate pace, with light to moderate pressure.

The athlete should be encouraged to refrain from unnecessary talk during the session, to focus on diaphragmatic breathing, to relax the body part being massaged, and to let go of any tensions felt. A massage session is a good opportunity for an athlete to develop relaxation skills.

A relaxing environment is quiet and warm, has indirect lighting, and minimizes distractions. A whirlpool, sauna, steam, or hot shower before the massage can also enhance its relaxing effects.

9. Tennis Elbow

Tennis elbow involves strain to the attachments of the wrist extensor muscles at the lateral epicondyle of the humerus. It is also called lateral epicondylitis. Onset of tennis elbow is usually gradual, brought on by overuse rather than by sudden trauma. As with any strain or tendinitis condition, there will be pain at the specific injury site (i.e., point tenderness at the lateral epicondyle of the humerus) with active-resisted muscle testing. Swelling, tightness, and discomfort along the involved muscle are also common.

Even with a diagnosis of tennis elbow, the massage practitioner should check for possible contraindications for massage. The elbow should not be catching or locking, have numbness or tingling, or exhibit significant restriction in the passive range of motion.

Treatment for tennis elbow usually begins with ice therapy and anti-inflammatory drugs to reduce inflammation and edema. Modification of activity and resting the affected arm is important at this stage. The tennis player can use this time to concentrate on other aspects of the game such as footwork and aerobic conditioning.

Massage used in the treatment of tennis elbow involves kneading to relieve tension in the muscles of the forearm and deep transverse friction of the tendons near their point of attachment. Begin the session with massage of the entire upper extremity with sliding strokes from wrist to shoulder, and gentle kneading and compression to increase local circulation and warm tissues.

A sliding movement variation called *draining* is then applied to the forearm. Figure 3.8 shows this technique with the athlete lying on a massage table in the supine position. The upper arm is resting on the table while you hold the forearm at a 45-degree angle. Encourage the athlete to relax the forearm muscles. While one hand holds the athlete's arm near the wrist, the active hand performs a deep sliding movement from wrist to elbow. The feel of the technique is one of draining the fluid in the forearm toward the elbow. Repeat the sliding motion all the way around the forearm. This technique may cause pain in tight muscles and should be applied within the comfort zone of the athlete. Use an even, steady pace.

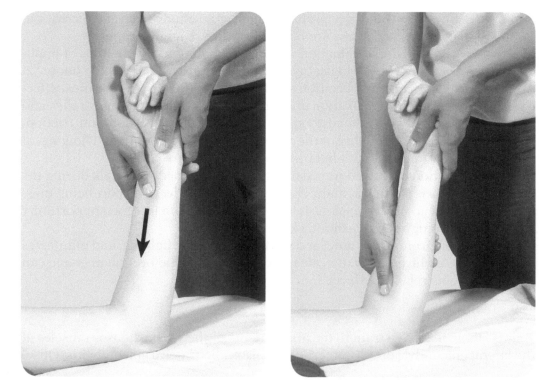

Figure 3.8 Draining—a deep sliding stroke to the forearm.

Extend the arm, resting it on the table with the forearm in pronation (i.e., palm down). Perform thumb slides to the extensor muscles, applying deep pressure as you slowly slide along the length of the muscles and their attachments. This action broadens the muscles. There will be pain as you pass over the tendons at the elbow. (For information on locating specific muscles, refer to Biel, 2001.)

To add active movement, ask the athlete to flex and extend at the wrist as you perform the thumb sliding technique. The wrist movement should be slow and steady. You can also apply digital pressure with active movement. Place your thumb on a tight place in the muscle and have the athlete flex and extend at the wrist. Move to another tense spot and repeat. This is effective near and at the tendon site.

The tendons are now ready for the application of deep transverse friction. This is best combined with ice massage. Perform ice massage to the lateral elbow for about 8 to 10 minutes prior to applying deep friction. During treatment you can periodically take a break to apply one minute of ice massage. This will help reduce the discomfort level of the athlete, as well as reduce inflammation.

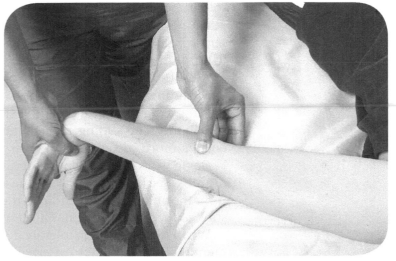

Deep transverse friction is most effective when applied to a tendon on stretch. To place the extensor tendons in an optimal position for friction, have the athlete lie in a supine position, place the upper extremity in an internally rotated position so that the extensor muscle tendons are now anterior, fully extend the elbow so that the arm is straight, and flex the wrist as shown in figure 3.9.

Figure 3.9 Deep transverse friction to attachments at the lateral epicondyle of the humerus in treatment for tennis elbow.

Apply deep transverse friction on and around the extensor muscle attachments with the thumb or fingertips. Friction is always painful with tendinitis and should be followed by comforting and soothing sliding techniques. End the session with ice massage, and have the athlete perform about 60 seconds of gentle active movement at the wrist. The entire session lasts from 15 to 30 minutes.

10. Tibialis Muscle Strain (Shin Splints)

Anterior and posterior tibialis strain is the most common cause of the pain that athletes call shin splints. *Shin splints*, which has become a catch-all term for pain in the anterior lower leg associated with physical activity, may actually be caused by several different conditions. Exercise-induced conditions that manifest as shin splints also include stress fracture of the tibia, tibial periostitus, microtears in the interosseous membrane, and compartment syndrome. In severe cases, a doctor's diagnosis is necessary to pinpoint the actual problem and rule out contraindications for massage.

Tibialis muscle strain is typically caused by a sudden increase in activity level, playing on hard surfaces, or lengthy endurance training. Reaction to such activities may escalate quickly from mild tightness to a muscle strain or tendinitis condition. The three levels of this condition are mild (pain is felt only after activity), moderate (pain is felt both before and after activity), and severe (pain is fairly consistent and the athlete stops or modifies activity in response).

Shin pain caused by anterior and posterior tibialis strain is felt on either side of the tibia bone, but not on the bone itself. Discomfort is felt along the length of the muscles rather than in one specific spot. If pain is spot specific or on the bone itself, refer the athlete for further diagnosis.

The treatment plan for tibialis muscle strain begins with modification of activity and rest, ice, and anti-inflammatory medication. Massage can then be applied to aid in restoration and healing.

Start the massage session with the athlete in the prone position with a bolster under the ankles. Warm and relax the entire upper and lower leg using full-palmar sliding strokes. Then focus on the lower leg, applying deeper strokes as the tissues soften and adding gentle kneading and compression. If the athlete is tolerating these techniques well, thumb slides using moderate pressing may be added. Apply friction to the Achilles tendon, and gently stretch the whole posterior muscle group including the gastrocnemius and soleus muscles. Spend 5 to 10 minutes on the posterior leg.

After the athlete turns over to a supine position, warm the entire anterior leg with sliding strokes using light to moderate pressure. Then focus on the lower leg, applying full-palmar sliding strokes and avoiding pressure directly over the shin bone. The sliding movements warm the tissues and prepare the area for deeper, more specific techniques.

Begin work on the tibialis anterior (TA) using a broadening technique with your thumbs (see figure 2.13) along the length of the muscle. Follow with thumb slides from the ankle to the knee along the TA. Begin gently and gradually increase pressure as the tissues soften. The goal is to eventually apply deep thumb slides.

When the athlete can tolerate deep thumb slides, apply them with active movement. Ask the athlete to alternately plantar-flex and dorsiflex the foot slowly as you perform the deep thumb slides on the TA muscle. For best results, remain in the optimal therapy zone (OTZ) of pressure and discomfort as explained in chapter 6. If you discover a specific area of congestion in the tissue, use deep transverse friction to the site.

Prior massage of the posterior leg and work on the tibialis anterior have increased local circulation and warmed tissues so that specific techniques can now be applied to the tibialis posterior (TP) muscle. Start with multiple-digit compression, which is applied with all eight fingers along the medial edge of the tibia. Sink into the soft tissues and back behind the bone to palpate the TP muscle. This technique requires finger strength and extremely short fingernails, as well as the cooperation of the athlete. Allow the athlete's feedback to guide how much pressure to use. Gradually increase pressure in a series of three to four applications.

Try applying the multiple-digit compression with the athlete alternately plantar-flexing and dorsiflexing the foot slowly. Friction can be applied by making small movements with your fingertips as you apply the digital pressure. When finished with these specific techniques, smooth over the area with sliding strokes. Apply ice to the shin and proceed to the foot.

Massage for shin splints should include the foot. Use sliding techniques to warm tissues on the dorsal and plantar sides of the foot. If any tight or congested areas are detected, apply circular friction. The TP muscle has numerous places of attachment on the bottom of the foot, including at the calcaneous, navicular, cuboid, cuneiform, and third and fourth metatarsal bones. The TA muscle tendon attaches at the first cuneiform and first metatarsal bones. All of these attachments should be checked for tenderness and adhesions, and deep friction applied as necessary.

The entire session devoted to shin splints can be completed in 30 minutes. Aggressive massage applications like this should not be overdone. Too much deep work on an injured site can result in increased inflammation or bruising.

Repeat the treatment every three to five days until the athlete can resume a moderate activity level. If no positive results are evident after the second massage session, consider referring the athlete back to a physician for further evaluation.

A complete treatment plan for shin splints includes correcting the factors that caused the condition in the first place. These might involve excessive foot pronation, inadequate footwear, too short adaptation time to new training levels, or changes in the playing or running surface. Although the massage practitioner can help, the entire sports health team needs to be part of a comprehensive treatment and prevention strategy.

11. Plantar Fascitis

Plantar fascitis is an inflammation of the plantar fascia on the sole of the foot. The primary role of this band of connective tissue is to support the foot's longitudinal arch. It is also called the plantar aponeurosis. Plantar fascitis causes severe pain on the sole of the foot. The condition may be caused by a sudden blow, or may be related to overuse, inadequate arch support, a hard playing surface, or tight shortened muscles in the lower leg.

An athlete with plantar fascitis experiences pain on the sole of the foot when using it after prolonged rest, such as first thing in the morning. There may be a tender spot on the heel at the point of attachment. If left untreated, a bone spur may develop causing heel spur syndrome. Foot muscles may also spasm from the pain associated with plantar fascitis.

As with the other examples of sports injury treatment, inflammation must first be addressed with ice, rest, and anti-inflammatory drugs. Because plantar fascitis is located on the sole of the foot, athletes cannot rest the area while continuing sports activity.

Self-care for plantar fascitis includes reducing activity that causes pain, using a longitudinal arch support, wearing shoes with adequate support, and avoiding going barefoot. An athlete can do a few minutes of self-massage on the foot before getting out of bed in the morning, and can use a tennis ball or golf ball for applying pressure to the sole of the foot during the day. A stretching regimen for the lower leg muscles can also help relieve stress on the sole.

Massage treatment for plantar fascitis begins with sliding strokes and other warming techniques applied to both the dorsal and plantar foot surfaces. For this example, the athlete will be in the supine position. Start very lightly, and increase pressure as the athlete's pain tolerance permits. Allow the massage to sooth the foot and coax the athlete into letting go of tension. Begin by using broad surfaces for sliding such as the palms or soft fist, and apply finger and thumb slides as tissues become less sensitive. The slides are applied in a longitudinal direction from the heel to the ball of the foot. Avoid too much pressure over tender spots.

If the condition allows for more aggressive therapy, deep transverse friction can be applied across the tissue. Be sensitive to the athlete's pain tolerance, but know that some pain is necessary for therapeutic results. A mere 60 seconds of deep transverse friction can make a significant difference in treating plantar fascitis. Finish with gentle sliding.

12. Before and After Surgery

Many disabling conditions are treated conservatively prior to resorting to surgery. Conservative treatment may include rest, exercises, hydrotherapy, electrical stimulation, medication, and other nonsurgical interventions.

Massage can be used to provide a better environment for other modalities used in conservative treatment. For example, massage may be applied to reduce muscle spasm in the lower back to enhance the effects of a traction device used for a spinal disc problem. Massage is often used as an adjunct to chiropractic treatment.

If surgery is needed after all, the athlete may have a more positive attitude toward the surgery if she feels satisfied that other avenues have been tried. Attitude is an important component of healing and recovery, and the relationship that develops between an athlete and her therapists can help reduce presurgery anxiety and be part of mental and emotional preparation for the procedure.

Massage may be especially beneficial to prepare the tissues and increase postsurgery recovery potential. For example, massage can improve circulation, reduce muscle tension and spasm, and reduce protective muscle splinting. This provides healthier, more pliable, and nutrient- and oxygen-rich tissue prior to surgery, and perhaps could improve subsequent tissue healing.

Enough evidence of the efficacy of massage exists to consider including massage in a conservative treatment program for many conditions. It is also beneficial to consider when surgery is scheduled weeks in advance.

Massage After Surgery: Acute Phase.   In the acute postsurgical phase, massage can be used to reduce edema in the surrounding tissues, improve general circulation and cell nutrition, reduce muscle spasm, and provide an analgesic effect. General circulatory and relaxation massage can reduce anxiety and mitigate some of the negative effects of inactivity.

Massaging the injury site directly, or if infection is present or highly likely, is contraindicated in the acute phase. There is a risk of doing more harm than good following surgery, so massage must be applied with utmost caution and care. Once the scar has healed and rehabilitation has begun, more aggressive massage may be applied.

Massage After the Acute Phase.   Past the acute phase, when sutures have been removed and healing is well underway, massage is indicated for restoration. In addition to general circulatory and relaxation benefits, massage encourages movement, reduces soreness, helps in the formation of healthy scar tissue, serves as reward motivation, and generally increases an athlete's sense of normality and well-being.

As discussed in chapter 1, massage promotes healthy scar formation, which is always a concern after surgery. Deep transverse friction is the most common technique for this purpose and may reduce the risk of reinjury or prevent the development of chronic pain at the incision site.

According to Arnheim and Prentice (1993), "When an injured body is immobilized for a period of time, a number of disuse problems adversely affect muscle, joints, ligaments, bone, and the cardiovascular system." They also said, "Whenever possible, the athlete, without aggravating the injury, must continue to exercise the entire body." (p. 348)

Massage can support the athlete's getting back in action sooner. It reduces muscle tension and pain and encourages movement. Recovery massage can be given after rehabilitation "workouts" to help reduce their negative effects. Patients may view massage as a reward for good effort on the rehabilitation equipment.

The psychological effects of massage enhance healing. Massage reduces anxiety over the outcome of the surgery and future athletic potential. In addition, the one-on-one attention, the time spent listening, and the caring touch expressed during massage promotes a greater sense of well-being, a more positive mental outlook, and perhaps a faster return to peak performance.

Chapter 4 describes applications of sports massage at athletic events. Sports massage is used to help athletes prepare for and recover from the rigors of competition.

STUDY QUESTIONS

1. What are the three restorative applications of sports massage?
2. When is massage for recovery given, and what are its goals?
3. How does a remedial session differ from a recovery session?
4. How do remedial massage applications and rehabilitation massage applications differ?
5. How does the massage application for chronic muscle tension differ from that for acute muscle tension?
6. What are the two types of postexercise soreness, and what are the primary goals of sports massage for this condition?
7. How is massage applied to reduce edema?
8. How is massage used to treat subclinical tendinitis?
9. What are the three grades of muscle strain? How is massage used in the treatment at each grade?
10. How is massage used with other modalities to treat a moderate sprain?
11. How can active movement be used with massage in the treatment of tennis elbow?
12. What techniques are used to massage the posterior tibialis muscle in the treatment of shin splints?
13. Why is an athlete's pain tolerance an important factor in treating plantar fascitis and other painful conditions?
14. How is massage used before and after surgery to enhance tissue repair?

SPORTS MASSAGE AT ATHLETIC EVENTS

LEARNING OUTCOMES

1. Explain the benefits of sports massage at athletic events.
2. Contrast the goals of pre-, inter-, and postevent massage.
3. Identify techniques appropriate for pre-, inter-, and postevent massage.
4. List the guidelines for pre-event sports massage.
5. List the guidelines for interevent sports massage.
6. List the guidelines for postevent massage.
7. Describe symptoms of, and first aid for, hyper- and hypothermia.
8. Describe five different techniques for relieving muscle cramps.

EVENT SPORTS MASSAGE

Sports massage is given at competitions to prepare athletes physically and mentally for events, to reduce the potential for injury, and to facilitate recovery after or between performances. Event sports massage is typically given by a massage specialist, a coach or trainer, or athletes themselves using self-massage techniques.

How sports massage is used at events varies with the type of event, the needs of the athletes, the facilities available, and the makeup of the athletes' support team. Types of sport events include games, meets, tournaments, races, or exhibitions. Sports massage specialists may be hired by the event organizers, may work for and travel with a specific team, or may provide massage to private client athletes. Competitions in individual sports lend themselves to all phases of event massage, but in team sports, the pregame and half-time warm-up routines usually preclude pre- and interevent massage.

Pre-, inter-, and postevent massage vary in their goals and in the techniques used. The needs of athletes before they perform are much different from their needs after the competition.

PRE-EVENT SPORTS MASSAGE

Readiness is the key word in pre-event sports massage. In the four hours preceding competition, massage can help prepare the body, mind, and spirit for the upcoming challenge. Its application may be as simple as the athlete frictioning his own legs as part of a warm-up routine, or may involve a short session with a sports massage specialist.

On the physical level, the goals of pre-event massage include increasing circulation to bring oxygen to the muscles (i.e., create *hyperemia*), warming connective tissue, reducing excessive muscle tension, and stretching for optimal range of motion. Mental and emotional goals are to improve mental clarity and focus and reduce precompetition anxiety. Massage may be part of an athlete's preparation ritual. As the body and mind of the whole athlete approach top functioning, performance potential increases.

To the extent that pre-event massage prepares muscles and other tissues for the stress that will be placed on them in the upcoming competition, it decreases injury potential. By contributing to warm-up and relieving muscle tension, massage helps prevent muscle pulls and tears.

In pre-event massage, care is taken to avoid eliciting any pain response. The point is to help the athlete feel ready to compete, not to remind him of that sore elbow.

Pre-Event Self-Massage

Athletes can use self-massage in a warm-up routine as a valuable complement to stretching. Massage techniques such as compression, circular friction, and percussion are easily self-administered and help prepare tissues for action. They increase local circulation and improve the pliability of connective tissues. Thumb pressure to stress points on tendons, and on certain acu-points, help make tissues suppler and more easily stretched (Meagher, 1990; Namikoshi, 1985). Light, rapid percussion stimulates nerves and improves alertness.

Self-Massage for Feet and Legs

Athletes can easily incorporate self-massage techniques into their warm-up routines. Self-massage for the legs is especially beneficial for runners, cyclists, tennis and basketball players, and martial artists. As in all pre-event sports massage, the pressure is light to moderate and the pacing is brisk. Athletes can use the following self-massage techniques for the legs and feet:

Hips (standing)

o Fist compressions and superficial friction to the buttocks muscles
o Thumb pressure along the iliac crest and around the head of the femur

Upper Leg (sitting)

o Superficial friction with knuckles to the thigh (medial and lateral)
o Palmar compression to quadriceps
o Jostling of the quadriceps
o Percussion of entire thigh (medial and lateral)

Lower Leg (sitting)

o Circular friction around the ankle
o Kneading the calf muscles
o Friction with the heel of the hand, and thumb pressure along tibialis anterior (lateral to shin bone)
o Circular friction around the knee (see figure 4.1)

Feet (sitting)

o Squeezing the entire foot
o Sliding and thumb pressure to the bottom of the foot
o Sliding to the top of the foot
o Percussion with fist to the bottom of the foot
o Mobilizing all of the joints in the foot

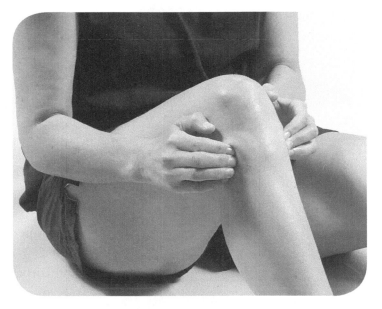

Figure 4.1 Self-massage—friction to the muscle attachments around the knee.

Pre-Event Partner Massage

Athletes can use some simple yet effective massage techniques with each other as warm-up before competition. The advantages of partner massage are that some areas of the body can be reached more easily by someone else (e.g., the upper back), the giver often has better leverage to exert more pressure, and athletes avoid stressing their own muscles. Anxiety-reducing effects are better if the massage is given by another sympathetic person.

Partner massage requires the cooperation of the two athletes and some sensitivity on the part of the giver. Using too much pressure and being too rough are common novice mistakes. The giver should respond to feedback from the athlete to "lighten up" or use more pressure. Partner massage is best learned well before a competition and under the supervision of a massage specialist.

The no-oil partner massage described in this section is given over clothing and in the lying or seated position. Athletes can be in one of several locations such as the training room, hallway, locker room, courtside, or in the stands. Partner massage can be given prior to athletes' regular warm-up and stretching routines, after a warm-up while waiting to be called for an event, at half-time, or between events.

Partner massage techniques for the shoulders and arms are beneficial for athletes in sports that require a lot of upper body activity—for example, swimmers, power lifters, tennis players, or gymnasts on parallel bars. The pressure should be light to moderate and the pacing brisk. Following is a sample partner massage for the upper body with the athlete sitting.

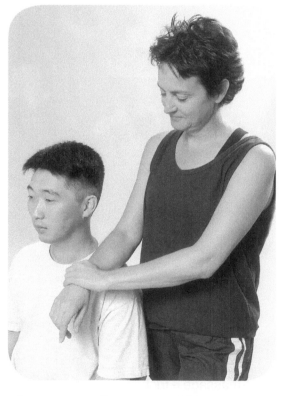

Figure 4.2 Partner massage—compression on the shoulder using the forearm.

Shoulders

○ Forearm compressions on the upper trapezius (see figure 4.2)

○ Thumb pressure along upper trapezius

○ Kneading the shoulders

Arm

○ Kneading the upper and lower arm muscles

○ Superficial friction (knuckles) to the entire arm

○ Jostling the arm

○ Gently squeezing the hand

Back

○ Superficial friction to paraspinal muscles (avoid the spine)

○ Direct elbow pressure to points on upper back

○ Percussion on shoulders and upper back

Pre-Event Massage by Coaches

Coach-to-athlete pre-event massage uses the same techniques as partner massage. Because team coaches are not likely to have time to spend with an individual athlete, they may use only a few simple techniques with a few players.

A coach experienced in palpation can assess the condition of specific tissues that may need extra warm-up or a trip to the athletic trainer for some last-minute treatment or taping. This is most likely an individual sport scenario.

Coaches may also use massage in much the same way that they use a slap on the back or hand on the shoulder to make physical contact to reassure an athlete before a performance. Massage provides an opportunity to give acceptable nonthreatening touch while offering verbal encouragement or last-minute instruction.

Pre-Event Massage by a Sports Massage Specialist

Massage specialists have advanced knowledge and skill in sports massage applications. They offer additional psychosocial support and complement the work of coaches, athletic trainers, and other sport professionals. They have the time to give pre-event massage when others are busy in different roles.

Sports massage specialists may give pre-event massages to athletes they have worked with for years, and with whom they have developed close relationships. As they are integrated into the athletes' support team, they also work closely with

---

HISTORY BRIEF 5

Massage Before and After Exercises in Ancient Rome c. 150 c.e.

Galen, the famous Roman doctor, was once a physician to the gladiators. He was also familiar with massage used by *aleiptes*, or anointers, and *paidotribes*, or trainers, to prepare athletes for their exercises and for recovery afterward.

In writing about massage before exercises, called *tripsis paraskeuastike*, Galen said,

> It is proper, by moderate rubbing with a linen cloth, to warm the whole body beforehand, and then to rub with oil . . . and one should at first rub quietly, and afterwards gradually increasing it, push the strength of the friction so far as evidently to compress the flesh but not to bruise it . . . for we do not rub so as to harden the body of the boy, whom we are training for the exercises, but to excite it to activity and augment its tone, and contract its porousness.

Galen gave instructions to apply rubbing all over the body and in all directions "in order that all the fibers of the muscles, as completely as possible, may be rubbed."

Galen believed that massage after exercises, called *apotherapeia*, helped remove the "residue of the excretions, warmed and rendered thin by exercises" which "remain locked up in the solid parts of the body" causing fatigue. About massage after exercises, he wrote, "but since the rubbing must be [neither] slow nor hard, we must pour oil plentifully over the body . . . for this contributes to both the quickness and softness of the rubbing . . . for it relaxes tension and softens the parts that have suffered in the more violent kinds of exertions." (Translations from *The Anatriptic Art* by Johnson, 1866)

coaches and trainers. For example, the trainer may ask the sports massage specialist to give special attention to an athlete returning after rehabilitation, or the coach may ask the sports massage specialist to give extra warming and stretching to certain muscles in a given athlete to improve performance potential.

At races and tournaments, sports massage specialists may also be called on to massage athletes whom they have never met before. When the athlete is a stranger, the practitioner must plan the session on the spot with little background information. He must rely on the athlete to identify what he needs and use his own palpation skills for information about the athlete's condition.

A typical pre-event session includes a combination of compression, digital pressure, circular friction, percussion, and joint mobilizing and stretching applied to all major muscle groups. This general massage is followed by work specific to the muscles and joints that will be used most in the upcoming event.

Experts generally agree that pre-event sports massage should do the following:

- Be short—15 to 20 minutes
- Have an upbeat tempo
- Avoid causing pain
- Concentrate on major muscle groups to be used in the upcoming performance
- Use techniques to increase circulation and ease of joint movement (e.g., compression, digital pressure, circular friction, broadening, percussion, jostling, joint mobilizing, and stretching)
- Adjust for mental and emotional readiness (e.g., be soothing for an anxious athlete and stimulating for most others)

Experienced massage practitioners may make exceptions to these guidelines to meet the needs of individual athletes. For example, athletes who receive massage frequently may want a deeper massage with attention to painful stress points. Other athletes may request a longer session; for example, a session four hours before an event may last 45 minutes instead of 15 minutes because it would not be part of the actual warm-up for an immediate performance.

INTEREVENT SPORTS MASSAGE

When an athlete is required to compete several times during a one- or two-day period (e.g., at a track meet) or continuously over a several-day period (e.g., in a cross-country bicycle race), interevent sports massage helps in both recovery and readiness. Interevent sports massage combines aspects of pre-event and postevent applications because the athlete is recovering from one bout and preparing for the next at the same time.

Interevent sessions are generally short and light with some variation depending on the proximity of the next performance. They focus on areas needing immediate attention. Specific goals depend on the unique needs of the individual athlete and on the nature of the sport.

Improving circulation for metabolite removal and better cell nutrition is a priority. Less invasive techniques (e.g., joint mobilizing, stretching, and positional release) are useful for tight areas. As in all event situations, deep and painful massage techniques should be avoided.

Interevent massage should do the following:

○ Be short—10 to 15 minutes

○ Focus on the recovery of the muscle groups used most

○ Relax specific areas of tension from the preceding performance

○ Use techniques to increase circulation and ease of joint movement (e.g., compression, digital pressure, circular friction, broadening, percussion, jostling, joint mobilizing, and stretching)

○ Adjust for mental and emotional readiness (e.g., be soothing for an anxious athlete and stimulating for most others)

○ Not be deep or painful

Exceptions to these recommendations can be made if the next event is several hours away (e.g., at a swim meet) or the next day (e.g., during a volleyball tournament or a five-day bicycle race). In the latter case, the massage session could last from 60 to 90 minutes and include general relaxation techniques.

In the special case of a very short time between events, simple recovery techniques (e.g., kneading) applied without oil may be used on the most stressed muscles. A familiar example of this is a trainer kneading a boxer's shoulders between bouts at a boxing match.

As in the pre-event situation, interevent massage may be given by a trainer, coach, another athlete, or the massage specialist. Self-massage is not as effective here because recovery massage applications are best received from someone else.

POSTEVENT SPORTS MASSAGE

Sports massage given within four hours after an event is focused on physical, mental, and emotional recovery. During postevent massage, injuries and other problems may be identified, evaluated, and referred for diagnosis if warranted. Minor injuries receive first aid or treatment when appropriate.

Guidelines for Postevent Massage

Postevent massage should do the following:

○ Be short (10 to15 minutes) if it occurs shortly after the last event, or longer (30 to 90 minutes) if it occurs an hour or more after the event

○ Feature lighter pressure, especially closer to the event time

○ Give specific attention to muscles stressed in the performance

○ Use techniques to flush out metabolites, reduce edema, relax tense muscles, and elicit the relaxation response (e.g., sliding strokes, compression, kneading, jostling, positional release, joint mobilizing, and stretches)

○ Include first aid or treatment for minor injuries

○ Include referral for injuries or conditions needing primary care attention

Before postevent massage, athletes should cool down to a normal heart rate, restore fluid and electrolyte balance, and do some light exercise such as walking. If there are suspected injuries that need evaluation, the athlete should be directed to an athletic trainer or physician before receiving massage.

Although self-massage can be beneficial in a postevent situation, the techniques used for recovery are more easily given by a partner, coach, or massage specialist. The athlete can also be more completely at rest during a massage given by someone else. Recovery massage techniques such as compression and kneading can be applied over a uniform or warm-up suit by a fellow athlete.

Postevent Role of the Sports Massage Specialist

The role of the massage specialist in the postevent situation includes both facilitating recovery and dealing with problem conditions. Whether or not treatment is offered for injuries depends on how close the massage session is to the actual performance, the severity of the injury, and the availability of other health professionals at the event. A massage given shortly after the event might include first aid, injury assessment, and referral for medical evaluation. Figure 4.3 shows an athlete receiving professional postevent massage.

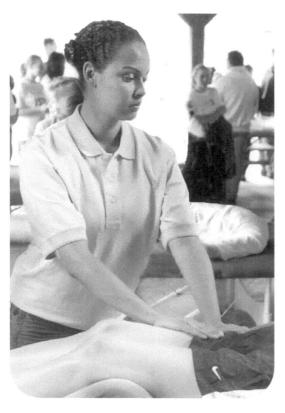

Figure 4.3 Athlete receiving postevent massage.

Injuries often seen in postevent situations include strains, sprains, muscle cramps, and bruising. Chafing from clothes rubbing on the skin may occur in distance events, as well as blisters on the feet. Although massage practitioners are generally at low risk for coming into contact with blood-borne pathogens, exposure to blood occasionally happens in postevent situations. Chafing, blood blisters, and road rash from falls are common at road races, triathlons, and cycling events. Appendix A describes sanitary precautions for sports massage at events.

Massage specialists should also be alert for signs of dehydration, hyperthermia, and hypothermia in the athlete. Water should be available for athletes to drink, blankets for warming, and ice for cooling down as well as for first aid and muscle cramping.

Aside from the need to give first aid for the occasional injury, the main focus of postevent massage is recovery. Techniques for recovery include light compression, sliding strokes, kneading, jostling, joint mobilizing, and stretching. Depth of pressure should be monitored carefully to avoid excessive compression of swollen tissues. Especially after long-distance events, muscles will be sore to the touch, therefore light flushing strokes should be used.

HYPERTHERMIA AND HYPOTHERMIA

Athletes may experience difficulty in maintaining a safe and comfortable core body temperature, particularly during long-distance events in extreme weather. When greeting athletes for postevent massage, you should assess their general condition and watch for signs of hyperthermia (i.e., overheating) and hypothermia (i.e., low body temperature). If you suspect either condition, give first aid immediately and refer the athlete for medical attention if the condition is severe.

Hyperthermia

Hyperthermia occurs when the core body temperature becomes dangerously high. The body's rate of heat production has exceeded its ability to dissipate the heat through normal heat-regulating mechanisms such as sweating. Conditions that increase the potential for hyperthermia include high air temperature (above 99 degrees), high humidity, high altitude, and dehydration.

Signs of hyperthermia are clumsiness, muscle cramps, stumbling, excessive sweating, no sweating, headache, nausea, dizziness, apathy, and impairment of consciousness. Loss of body fluids is a major factor in hyperthermia, and athletes should replace fluids adequately before receiving postevent massage. If athletes come for massage showing signs of hyperthermia, offer them more fluids. First aid should be given for the following conditions:

Muscle cramps. See the directions for treatment of muscle cramps in the following section. If an athlete begins to have cramping throughout the body, pack her in ice and get immediate medical attention.

Heat exhaustion. Symptoms of heat exhaustion include headache, nausea, hair erection on the chest and upper arms, chills, unsteadiness, fatigue, cool skin, and sweating. If an athlete shows signs of heat exhaustion, do the following:

○ Refer the athlete for medical attention.

○ While waiting for medical help, administer first aid including ice on the back of the neck, rest in the cool shade or in front of a fan, and cool fluids.

Heatstroke. Symptoms of heatstroke include incoherent speech, confusion, aggressive behavior, unconsciousness, and absence of sweating. If you suspect that an athlete has heatstroke, do the following:

○ Refer the athlete for medical attention immediately.

○ Do *not* administer fluids by mouth.

Hypothermia

Hypothermia, or having a core body temperature much below normal, occurs when the body's rate of heat production is less than its rate of heat loss. Conditions that increase the potential for hypothermia include cold, wet, or rainy weather and high altitude.

Early signs of hypothermia include shivering, euphoria, the appearance of intoxication, and blue lips and nail beds. As the core temperature continues to fall, the athlete will become disoriented and may hallucinate, become combative, or lose consciousness. If an athlete shows signs of hypothermia, do the following:

○ Refer the athlete for medical attention immediately; advanced hypothermia is a medical emergency.

○ While waiting for medical help, administer first aid by having the athlete change into dry clothes, drink warm fluids, wrap in a blanket, cover the head, and move around (e.g., walk or receive passive joint mobilizing).

RELIEVING MUSCLE CRAMPS

After the all-out effort of competition, especially in distance events, muscle cramping may occur. Dehydration can lead to muscle cramping, so before giving sports massage, be sure that athletes have replaced fluids and electrolytes lost by sweating. If cramping occurs during postevent massage, give the athlete more fluids. The following manual techniques are used to relieve muscle cramps. Cramping in the calf muscles is used for illustration.

Direct compression. Sustained pressure is applied to a muscle spasm with the full hand, fist, forearm, or knee. Take the muscle in spasm off stretch before applying pressure. See figure 4.4.

Mild static stretch. Apply a mild static stretch to the cramping muscle. See figure 4.5.

Reciprocal inhibition. Engage the antagonist to the cramping muscle in an isometric contraction, thereby triggering reciprocal inhibition and relaxation of the muscle in spasm. Follow this with a mild static stretch. See figure 4.6.

Approximation. Simulate muscle relaxation by grasping the belly of the muscle on both sides of the cramp, then pushing your hands toward each other and holding for 7 to 10 seconds. After the muscle relaxes, apply a mild static stretch. See figure 4.7.

Ice. Numb a cramping muscle with ice or ice massage, followed by a mild stretch. Ice is also useful after the muscle has relaxed to reduce soreness and facilitate continued relaxation. See figure 4.8.

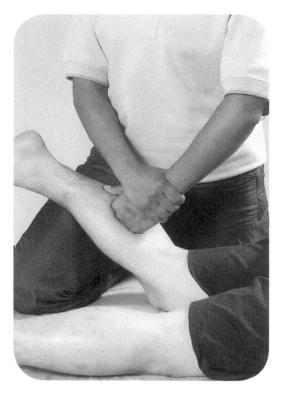

Figure 4.4 Direct compression used to relieve muscle cramp.

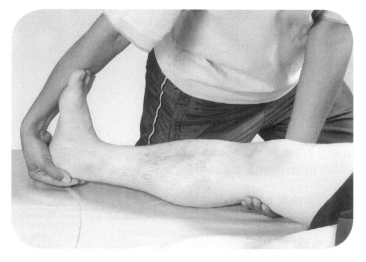

Figure 4.5 Mild stretch used to relieve muscle cramp.

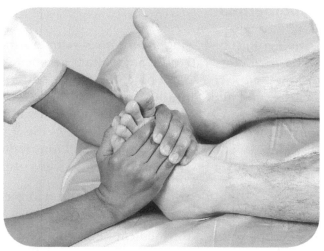

Figure 4.6 Reciprocal inhibition used to relieve muscle cramp.

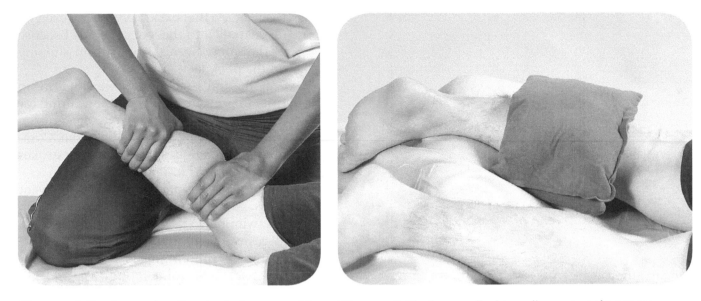

Figure 4.7 Approximation technique used to relieve muscle cramp.

Figure 4.8 Ice applied to relieve muscle cramp.

EVENT SPORTS MASSAGE AT A SWIM MEET

The swim meet offers a good example of how sports massage might be provided at individual sport events. The host school or event sponsor might arrange for sports massage to be available at the event and set aside a space so that swimmers can receive pre-, inter-, and postevent massage as needed.

Some teams also travel with their own sports massage specialists. The following paragraphs describe how an athletic department can provide sports massage for its swim team at away meets (Jill Bielawski, former massage therapist for the University of Arizona swim team, personal interview, September 2, 1993).

Pre-Event Sports Massage at a Swim Meet

The team typically arrives two days before an important meet to give the swimmers time to settle into their new surroundings. A massage room is set up at the team's hotel, and swimmers receive full-body massages that last from 30 to 60 minutes to help them calm down and begin to prepare for the meet. The massage specialist employs moderately firm pressure and addresses trigger points, but does not use deep techniques (e.g., deep transverse friction).

At the meet site, an area near the pool is usually set aside for massage tables. See figure 4.9. On event day, the pre-event massage usually lasts from 10 to 20 minutes. Its purpose is to help the swimmers get mentally prepared, focused, and psyched-up, and to enhance the warm-up by increasing general circulation. Images invoked include "getting things moving," feeling "as light as air," and "fluffing up" the muscles. Many believe that preparation for a competitive swimmer is about 50 percent mental, and pre-event massage helps in that process.

Pre-event massage for swimmers uses fast-paced sliding strokes, jostling, joint mobilizing, and stretches. Light oil may be applied to the torso, arms, and legs because "many swimmers like the feel of oil on their bodies—like gliding through

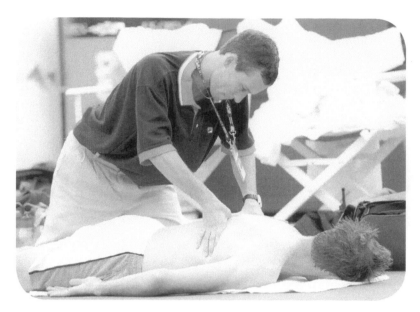

Figure 4.9 Event massage at a swim meet.

the water." (Bielawski, 1993) However, no oil is applied to the feet or hands because of the safety hazard posed from slipping on the pool deck or blocks.

Sometimes swimmers wear warm-up suits to prevent chilling while waiting for their events. In this case, massage is given over the clothing and no oil is used. Compression techniques replace sliding strokes for increasing circulation.

The areas of concentration in pre-event massage for swimmers vary depending on the swimmer's specific event. For example, in a pre-event massage for a freestyle swimmer, the emphasis is on the arms and back with joint mobilizing and hip stretches. For a swimmer specializing in the breaststroke, emphasis is on the arms, neck, back, and legs, particularly the adductors and abductors.

Interevent Sports Massage at a Swim Meet

Massage given between swimming events is short (10 to 15 minutes) and fast paced. It is most often performed over warm-up suits to prevent chilling, and therefore oil is not usually used. Care is taken to stimulate, *not* sedate, the swimmer. Compression, sliding strokes, and kneading on the arms and legs help keep muscles warm and enhance circulation.

Occasionally a muscle will have tightened up because of stress at the site of a previous injury. In that case, the massage may be deeper and more aggressive to relieve the restriction in movement and increase mobility. Ice may also be applied to relieve tension and soreness at the site.

Postevent Sports Massage at a Swim Meet

A postevent massage can be performed poolside over a sweat suit to prevent chilling, and lasts about 30 minutes. At this point swimmers may be emotionally or physically exhausted.

Massage specialists giving postevent massages at a swim meet use light compression, jostling, joint mobilizing and stretches, giving special attention to areas stressed most in the competition. Slower-paced massage facilitates general relaxation, which is appropriate at this point.

If postevent massage is given in the makeshift hotel massage room, it may be performed directly on the skin using oil. The swimmers are less exhausted and the hotel room can be kept warmer than the typical pool area. Sliding strokes and kneading will enhance general relaxation and increase circulation to flush out waste products and bring nutrients to tired muscles.

Between competitive events, athletes continue to train and practice their skills. Chapter 5 describes how to use maintenance sports massage between competitions to help athletes maintain optimal physical and mental condition.

STUDY QUESTIONS

1. How does pre-event massage help prepare athletes for competition?
2. What are the goals of pre-event sports massage, and what techniques are typically used to achieve them?
3. Why are certain types of techniques avoided in pre-event massage? What are they?
4. How can an athlete use self-massage to warm up her legs?
5. What are common mistakes of novice massage providers, and how can they be avoided when athletes give massage to each other?
6. Which no-oil techniques can athletes use to give each other pre-event massage of the upper body?
7. How are the general guidelines for pre-, inter-, and postevent massage similar? How do they differ?
8. Should an athlete come for massage soon after an event? What should he do before receiving postevent massage?
9. What types of injuries are massage specialists likely to see when giving postevent massage? When do they refer the athlete for medical evaluation?
10. What are the signs of hyperthermia? What are the appropriate first aid measures?
11. What are the signs of hypothermia? What are the appropriate first aid measures?
12. How are good sanitation practices applied in event sports massage?

CHAPTER 5

MAINTENANCE SPORTS MASSAGE

LEARNING OUTCOMES

1. List the goals of maintenance sports massage.
2. Explain the guidelines for maintenance massage sessions.
3. Identify common problem areas for athletes in different sports.
4. Describe a maintenance session using oil.
5. Describe remedial applications for different body regions.

OVERVIEW OF MAINTENANCE SPORTS MASSAGE

Maintenance sports massage refers to massage received by athletes on a regular basis as part of their training regimen. The purpose of maintenance massage is to help athletes maintain optimal physical condition and address problem areas as they arise during training and the competitive season.

To accomplish these goals, maintenance sessions include general recovery massage on the entire body with remedial applications in problem areas. Extra attention is given to tight or sore muscles, stiff joints, and former injury sites. Afterward, athletes should feel relaxed, loose, and refreshed.

Because the nature of maintenance massage is so individual, there is no "typical" session. Maintenance sessions focus on the specific needs of the athlete at a particular time in her training cycle. However, certain routines can be used as a starting point and modified as needed. During a basic routine, when a massage specialist comes to a section of the body with a problem condition, she should simply spend more time on that area using techniques designed to treat the specific problem.

Chapter 3 offers a good example of a basic recovery routine that does not use oil or other lubricant, and also some specific remedial massage applications. In this chapter we outline a general recovery routine that does use oil, integrating examples of remedial applications for different body regions. But first, some of the basic guidelines for maintenance sports massage, and some common problem areas will be discussed.

Maintenance sports massage should do the following:

- Be scheduled regularly with a massage specialist (i.e., once or twice weekly, or biweekly)
- Last from 60 to 90 minutes
- Include recovery massage as a foundation
- Include remedial massage applications for problem conditions
- Give extra attention to areas stressed in the athlete's sport
- Use a full range of massage techniques to achieve session goals
- Be moderate in tempo

COMMON PROBLEM AREAS

Before a maintenance session, athletes should identify problem areas both verbally and on a Trouble Spots Body Chart as explained in chapter 6. In addition, as the massage practitioner moves from area to area during a general maintenance massage, he will encounter areas that need more detailed attention. These usually involve tight, stiff, or sore muscles. Edema may be evident around certain joints. These problems commonly result from overstress or overuse, past injuries, or improper body mechanics.

Problem spots require additional time for recovery massage and specific remedial massage applications. Techniques well suited to address specific musculoskeletal problems include deep sliding strokes, circular and deep transverse fric-

HISTORY BRIEF 6

Postl Advertisement c. 1917

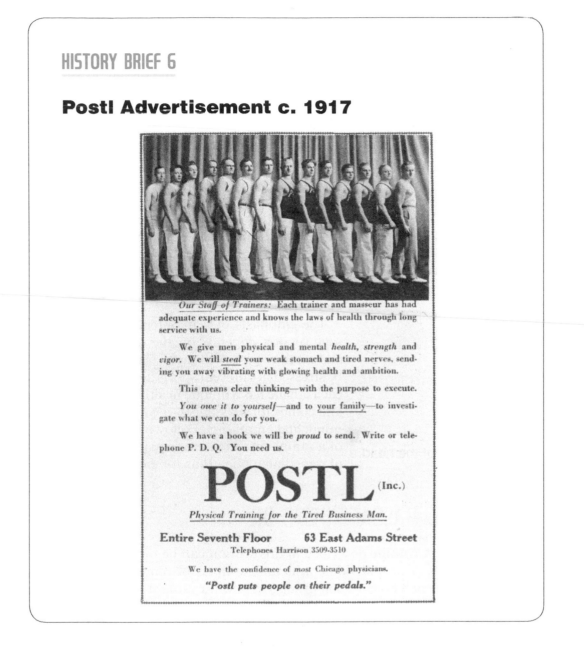

Our Staff of Trainers: Each trainer and masseur has had adequate experience and knows the laws of health through long service with us.

We give men physical and mental *health, strength* and *vigor.* We will *steal* your weak stomach and tired nerves, sending you away vibrating with glowing health and ambition.

This means clear thinking—with the purpose to execute.

You owe it to yourself—and to your family—to investigate what we can do for you.

We have a book we will be *proud* to send. Write or telephone P. D. Q. You need us.

POSTL (Inc.)

Physical Training for the Tired Business Man.

Entire Seventh Floor   63 East Adams Street
Telephones Harrison 3509-3510

We have the confidence of *most* Chicago physicians.

"Postl puts people on their pedals."

tion, trigger point therapy, digital pressure, and stretching. Light sliding strokes and lymphatic drainage massage are used to reduce swelling around joints.

Legs and Hips.   Athletes susceptible to leg and hip problems include runners, long and high jumpers, skiers, cyclists, martial artists, basketball players, and soccer players. Deep friction and digital pressure on tendons; kneading and broadening techniques; trigger point therapy; and stretching at the ankle, knee, and hip are often helpful.

Back.   Because both upper and lower body movements involve the back, athletes in most sports experience tension and soreness in this area. Deep sliding strokes, compression, circular friction, and digital pressure are easily applied to the large muscles of the back. The forearm and elbow can be used effectively to apply deep pressure to the back muscles.

Arms, Chest, and Shoulders. Athletes prone to upper body problems include gymnasts; tennis and other racket sport players; martial artists; golfers; and volleyball, baseball, and softball players. Certain field events such as discus, shot put, and javelin also stress the upper body. Deep friction and digital pressure on tendons, trigger point therapy, and stretching of the shoulder muscles address specific stressed areas. Compression, kneading, and broadening techniques relax muscles and increase local circulation.

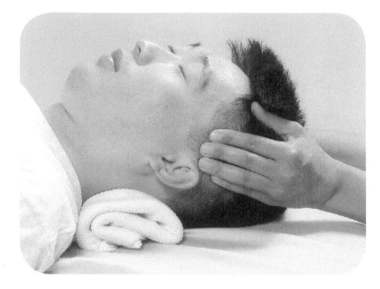

Figure 5.1 Circular friction to the sides of the head.

Neck and Head. The neck and head are sometimes forgotten as areas of tension except in sports such as wrestling and American football. Thumb slides, circular friction, and digital pressure along the upper trapezius and the posterior cervical muscles relieve tension in the area. Circular friction can be applied to the sides of the head and the forehead (see figure 5.1). Massage can relieve tension headaches caused by anxiety and stress.

The emphasis of a maintenance sports massage session depends on the individual athlete and on the sport. Although certain areas tend to be stressed in different sports as noted previously, each athlete has a unique health and injury profile and comes for massage as a whole person (body, mind, and emotions). Following is a description of a sample maintenance session with examples of remedial applications for each region.

MAINTENANCE MASSAGE USING OIL

The basic recovery routine described in this section can be modified to address the specific needs of an individual athlete. Examples of remedial applications are described for each body region to suggest how they might be integrated into the session.

Keep in mind that this is a general description only. It is impossible to describe every movement made during a massage session. No two sessions are exactly alike. The accomplished massage practitioner combines, blends, alternates, and otherwise varies movements to address specific conditions found in tissues and joints during a session. The qualities of movement (pace, rhythm, pressure) will also vary with the situation. Use this routine as a model for practicing general maintenance massage using oil.

This sample routine was designed for an athlete who filled out the Trouble Spots Body Chart shown in figure 5.2. Refer to chapter 6 for a description of the use of the chart.

Prone Position

The athlete should be laying facedown on a comfortable surface, preferably a massage table. Use a professional face cradle if available, or turn the head to the side. The athlete should be draped appropriately as in any standard massage

Figure 5.2

Trouble Spots Body Chart

Name *John Adams*   Date   *3-11-04*

Sport *Runner—Marathon*   Age *27*   Gender: (M) F

Current training intensity (circle one):   (Easy) Moderate High

Today's emotional stress level (circle one):   Low (Medium) High

Last competition *2-17-04*   Next competition *6-18-04*

Please identify your body's current trouble spots on the diagram below using the trouble spots key.

KEY: ○   circle areas of tightness
       ●   shaded circle for pain
       X   "X" over stiff joints
       ≋   wavy lines over areas of numbness or tingling
       #   hatch marks over recent bruises or wounds

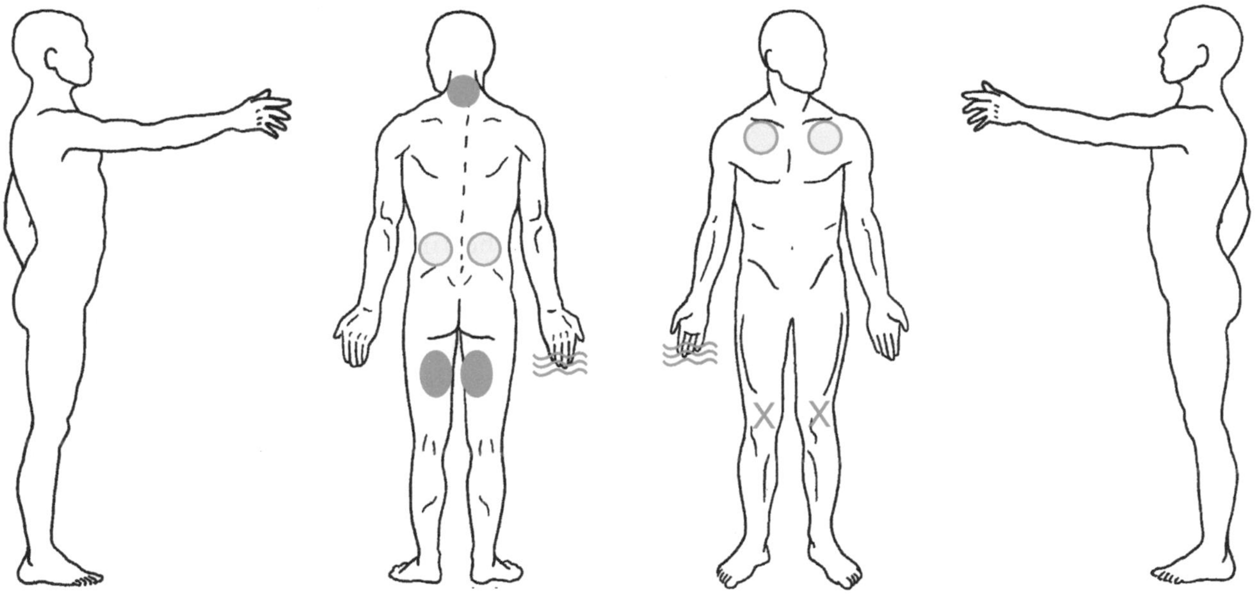

Comments   *3 wks since last marathon; 3 mos til next race.*

Tight lower back and neck; hamstrings feel tight; knees stiff;

need to relax—JA

session. A large towel is often used instead of a sheet for draping in sport settings. Place bolsters under the ankles and shoulders for comfort. Use good-quality massage oil and apply it sparingly as needed to facilitate sliding and avoid chafing the skin.

Back

First, warm the back with compressions applied over the drape, then undrape and apply oil with long sliding strokes from the shoulders to the waist. The hands are in full-palmar position to provide a broad contact surface. Be sure to include the sides as well as the muscles along the spine. Repeat several times, increasing pressure as tissues become warm.

Once the entire back is sufficiently warm and the skin begins to redden, proceed with more specific massage. Starting with the upper back, knead the upper trapezius and the whole area from the neck to the shoulder. Gently knead the muscles of the neck and apply sliding strokes with the fingers to the posterior neck muscles.

Then, work a bit more deeply between the shoulder blades using superficial friction with the knuckles over the rhomboids, followed by circular friction with the fingertips. Repeat the friction techniques to the muscles on the shoulder blades. Every so often perform some long, deep sliding strokes to the entire back, and return to the more specific friction techniques.

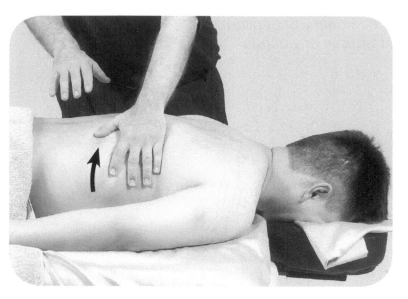

Figure 5.3 Full-palmar sliding stroke with spread fingers between the ribs.

Apply deep sliding strokes with the forearm to the erector muscles along the spine, from the shoulders to the waist. Do not put pressure on the spine, but keep to either side. Then apply circular friction along the length of the erector muscles. Transition with full-palmar strokes to the entire back.

Use deep sliding strokes to massage the sides of the thorax. The small spaces between the ribs can be contacted with the fingers spread. Use a sliding movement from lateral to medial, pulling up and around the sides of the back as shown in figure 5.3.

Apply thumb slides to the muscles between the pelvis and the ribs. Finish with full-palmar sliding strokes from the shoulders to the waist. Re-cover the back to keep it warm.

Remedial Application. Tightness in the lower back is a common complaint of athletes. It is described as a "band of tension" across the lumbar region. The origin of lower back tension is frequently found in the upper buttocks muscles, which can be easily addressed with the athlete in the prone position.

With the back muscles warm and relaxed, prepare the upper buttocks muscles using kneading, compressions, and sliding strokes. Once the buttocks area is warmed up, apply thumb slides laterally from the sacrum to the hip across the

HISTORY BRIEF 7

Gymnasia in Ancient Greece c. 300 B.C.E.

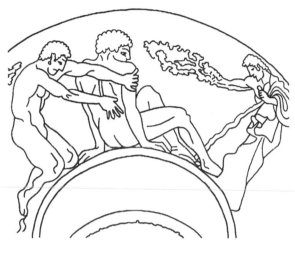

Some of the earliest records of massage for athletes are from the ancient Greek gymnasia. Elite athletes of the ancient Olympic Games, as well as ordinary citizens who went to the gymnasia, received massage as part of their training routines. Professional trainers called *paidotribes*, who were often retired athletes themselves, served as coaches, nutritionists, physiotherapists, and masseurs.

The routine at the ancient Greek gymnasia was described in *The Anatriptic Art* by Johnson (1866).

The youth was first rubbed by the *paidotribes* with oil; this process was called preparatory rubbing—*tripsis paraskeuastike*. He then proceeded to some of the lighter exercises, as playing at ball; after which he sprinkled himself with Egyptian dust, and sought a companion to wrestle with. When sufficiently exercised, he passed into the room of the anointer, *aleiptes*, who by aid of the stlengis or strigil, as the Romans called it, helped him to scrape off his dust, oil, and sweat, and then rubbed him again with oil, which process was called *apotherapeia*. This done, he entered the warm bath, and after a short stay proceeded to the cold bath, and from the cold bath he returned to the *aleiptes*, who anointed him a second time, and sent him about his business.

gluteus maximus, piriformis, and gluteus medius muscles. The knuckles or elbows can also be used to perform the sliding technique. Apply deeper pressure as the tissues soften. The intent is to stretch the muscles away from the sacrum.

Then, apply circular friction all along the iliac crest on the site of buttocks muscle attachments. Use single- or multiple-digit overlay to reinforce the fingers. Be cautious when applying deep techniques, especially single-digit techniques, to avoid harming the easily bruised adipose tissues of the buttocks region. Once the buttocks muscles have relaxed, go back and check the lumbar region for tightness in the lower back muscles.

Legs

Uncover the athlete's right leg and tuck the drape securely. Stand at the side of the table near the feet, facing the athlete's head. Begin with full-palmar sliding movements from ankle to hip. Deepen pressure as the tissues become warm. Apply most pressure as the hands slide from distal to proximal, and lighten contact as they return to the ankle for the next stroke. The idea is to push fluids mechanically toward the body cavity.

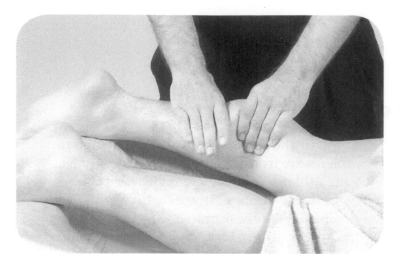

After the warm-up, massage the leg in parts from the hip to the ankle. Work the buttocks muscles first, then the posterior thigh, and then the lower leg. Apply compression, deep sliding strokes, broadening, circular friction, and kneading to increase circulation and relax the muscles in the area. Knead the muscles of the lower leg as shown in figure 5.4. Finish as you began with long sliding strokes from ankle to hip. Re-cover the leg. Repeat the sequence on the other side.

Figure 5.4 Kneading the muscles of the lower leg.

Remedial Application. If you notice greater tension on the medial side when performing sliding strokes on the back of the thigh, perform some additional sliding to assess the situation. This type of *active palpation* helps you evaluate the degree of tension and locate spots of tenderness. Ask the athlete, "Does that feel tight to you, is it sore, has it been bothering you lately?" (Note: This type of feedback is appropriate for maintenance sessions, but should be avoided in pre-event sessions to prevent planting the seeds for doubt or apprehension right before competition.) If you find a particular muscle such as the semimembranosus a little hypertonic, but not injured, you can work the muscle specifically to release tension.

To get the hamstring muscles into a loose and relaxed position, lift the athlete's lower leg off the table and place her ankle on your shoulder for support. Apply sliding strokes directly on the tense muscle from distal to proximal attachments. Increase the specificity of the application by changing from knuckle to single-digit to thumb placement as you deepen pressure.

Then place the leg back onto the table with a bolster under the ankle to extend the hamstring muscle group. Repeat the sliding strokes. If tension persists, but the muscle is not very painful, apply the sliding techniques with active movement (i.e., ask the athlete to flex and extend the leg slowly as you slide over the muscle).

This entire remedial application takes one to three minutes. You can devote more time to this trouble spot if needed, but if the athlete has other complaints, work quickly and effectively, and move on.

Supine Position

The athlete lays on his back with a bolster under the knees, and possibly a neck roll or pillow under the head, and is draped appropriately. Uncover the left leg.

Legs

Before applying lubricant, do some compressions to the thigh muscles. Rocking compressions not only relax the thigh muscles, but also mobilize and warm the hip joint and relax the entire leg. Then apply oil and warm the leg using full-palmar sliding strokes from ankle to hip.

After the warm-up, apply kneading and broadening techniques to the entire thigh. See figure 5.5. Finish and transition with sliding strokes to the whole leg.

To massage the lower leg, place the heels of the hands on either side of the shin bone, fingers around the calf muscles, and squeeze the muscles using the whole hand. Move from place to place from ankle to knee. Circular friction and broadening can also be applied with the heel of the hands. Perform thumb slides along the tibialis anterior, lateral to the shin. Finish and transition with sliding strokes to the whole leg.

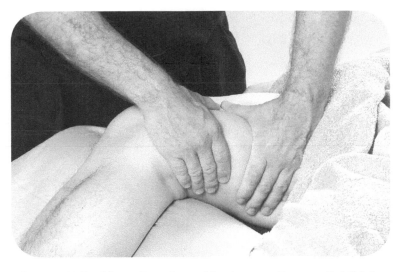

Figure 5.5 Kneading the adductors on the medial thigh.

Massage the ankle with circular friction using the heels of the hands or the fingertips. Then apply squeezing, sliding, and joint-mobilizing techniques to the foot. Figure 5.6 shows sliding movements applied to the dorsal foot. The fist can be used to apply sliding strokes to the soles of the feet.

Mobilize all the joints from the hip to the toes to conclude work on the leg. Re-cover the leg. Repeat the sequence on the right leg.

Remedial Application. You notice that the attachments of the thigh muscles feel a bit tight, or *congested*, near the knee. Deep transverse friction to the specific area of tightness helps increase the pliability of these connective tissues and breaks adhesions. Apply 20 to 30 seconds of deep transverse friction directly to the attachments, followed by palmar sliding to the entire thigh. The palmar sliding facilitates relaxation of the muscles involved and gives the athlete some relief from the painful friction techniques. Repeat the friction and sliding cycle two to three times to the same tissue, and then the whole cycle on other sites around the knee as needed.

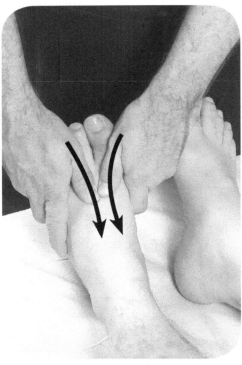

Figure 5.6 Sliding stroke with thumbs on the dorsal surface of the foot.

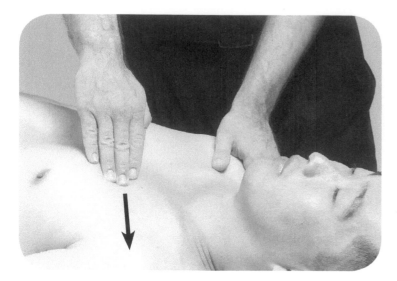

Figure 5.7   Multiple-digit sliding on the pectoral muscles.

Chest

Uncover the upper chest; however, keep women's breasts covered at all times. Massage the upper chest with sliding strokes on the pectoral muscles, or compression over the drape. Use your palm, fingertips, or fist (see figure 5.7). Begin with light pressure and gradually work deeper. Apply circular friction to muscle attachments. Do not massage into the breast tissue. Re-cover for warmth.

Remedial Application.   You notice that the athlete's shoulders are pulled forward, and he winces in pain as you palpate the pectoralis minor muscle. The muscle feels tight and ropey. Because this muscle is very sensitive when hypertonic, work slowly and ask the athlete for feedback on the amount of pressure you are using.

Once the area is warmed up, apply sliding strokes with the fingers or thumb directly over the pectoralis minor in the direction of the fibers. Repeat several times, increasing pressure as tension in the muscle eases. This broadens and stretches the muscle, encouraging relaxation. Finish with sliding strokes over the area using a broad surface such as a loose fist or palm, and stretch the muscle with the arm overhead.

Arm and Shoulder

Uncover the arm to the shoulder. Begin with the arm in pronation, palm down, on the table. Stand at the side facing the athlete's head. Apply oil to the entire arm from wrist to shoulder with palmar sliding strokes. Massage the upper arm and shoulder with sliding, kneading, broadening, and circular friction. Mobilize the shoulder with a wagging technique. Transition with sliding strokes to the whole arm.

Massage the forearm with deep palmar sliding, followed by thumb slides in parallel strips from wrist to elbow. Knead the forearm flexor and extensor muscles, and finish with more sliding strokes.

Hand massage is similar to foot massage, with sliding on both dorsal and palmar surfaces. Gently squeeze each finger, and then slide off as shown in figure 5.8. Finish the arm with joint-mobilizing techniques. Re-cover, and repeat on the other side.

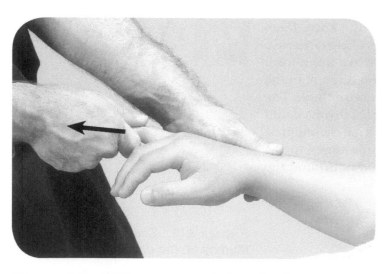

Figure 5.8   Sliding movement along the fingers.

Remedial Application.   The athlete complains of numbness in the last three fingers of the right hand, a symptom of nerve entrapment that can be caused by several different factors. In this case, refer the athlete to a primary health care provider for diagnosis. Many cases of nerve entrapment can be treated with massage, but the underlying cause must be determined. Diagnosis is outside of the scope of sports massage specialists.

Neck

Stand or sit at the athlete's head. Apply sliding strokes from the shoulder up the posterior and lateral neck to the head on both sides. Move the neck through a passive range of motion into lateral flexion, flexion, and rotation. Apply sliding strokes and circular friction along the posterior cervical muscles. Finish as you began with sliding from shoulder to head.

End with a slight traction of the neck as shown in figure 5.9. Hold the head in your palms, fingers grasping lightly under the occipital ridge. Pull gently back. Release the traction after about 15 seconds and continue to hold the head for another 10 seconds. Slowly pull your hands away to end the session.

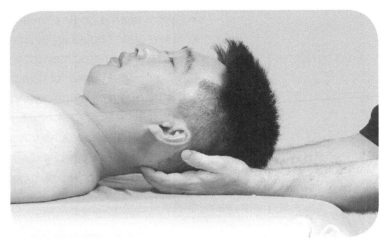

Figure 5.9 Slight traction to the neck.

Remedial Application. Common hot spots in the neck include the suboccipital region, levator scapula, anterior scalenes, and sternocleidomastoid (SCM) muscles. All of these spots can be treated with careful application of digital pressure and sliding techniques. Because the neck is relatively small on most people, the fingertips and thumb are often used to apply techniques to these muscles.

If you find tension and soreness in the sternocleidomastoid (SCM) muscles on both sides of the neck, suspect trigger points. A special application of compression or gentle squeezing or grasping can be used to treat the muscle with the client in the supine position (see figure 5.10).

Once the area is warmed up, grasp the middle of the SCM between the thumb and forefinger and gently squeeze it and pull it away from the tissues underneath. You can use a paper tissue between your hand and the skin to provide the traction needed for this technique. Be sure that you are touching only the muscle, and not other delicate structures in the area. Hold the pressure for about 10 seconds and then release. Repeat along the muscle as necessary. About five squeezes is usually enough to effect some relief from tension.

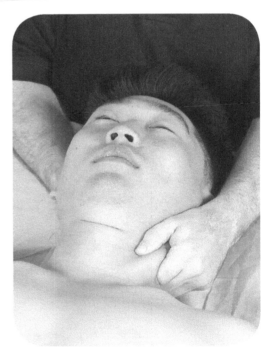

Figure 5.10 Squeezing the SCM to relieve tension and trigger points.

This can be a painful application, so communicate compassion to the athlete, while responding to his feedback on the pain involved in relieving trigger points. Such communication is essential in maintenance sports massage, not only for effective treatment of trouble spots, but also to build a good working relationship based on trust and understanding.

Maintenance sessions are the most comprehensive sports massage applications because they involve both recovery and remedial work. Chapter 6 explains in more detail how to plan and perform sports massage sessions to achieve athletes' goals.

STUDY QUESTIONS

1. What are the goals of maintenance sports massage?
2. How often should an athlete receive maintenance massage?
3. How long are maintenance sessions?
4. What is the benefit of using oil in a maintenance session?
5. Is there a typical maintenance sports massage session? Explain.
6. Which areas of the body are stressed in different sports?
7. Which massage techniques are best suited for warming an area?
8. Which massage techniques are used for specific therapeutic goals?
9. How do you know how much time to spend on each body section during maintenance massage?

CHAPTER 6

PLANNING AND GIVING SPORTS MASSAGE

LEARNING OUTCOMES

1. Describe the elements of planning a sports massage session.
2. Explain the use of the Trouble Spots Body Chart.
3. Understand the choice and sequence of technique applications relative to session goals.
4. Appreciate a routine approach to sessions.
5. Evaluate the use of sport-specific routines.
6. Compare topical substances used in sports massage.
7. Identify good body mechanics.
8. Describe important aspects of massage technique performance.
9. Understand how to use feedback from the athlete about pain.
10. Appreciate the importance of working in the optimal therapy zone for maximum therapeutic results.

SPORTS MASSAGE SESSIONS

Sports massage sessions are individualized and require some advanced planning. An experienced massage specialist can sketch a general plan quickly given key bits of information, but a student or beginner needs to think things out more carefully. This chapter addresses the essential elements of planning and giving a sports massage session.

Although a general plan can be made beforehand, many of the specific details of giving massage emerge during a session as the massage specialist interacts with the athlete verbally and physically. Qualities such as pressure, rhythm, pacing, and specificity are determined on the spot as the massage progresses. The details are altered as the receiver reacts to the massage and a clearer picture of what is called for evolves during the session.

In addition to the massage techniques themselves, practitioners must handle physical objects such as sheets, bolsters, towels, and bottles. These aspects of general mechanics and good body mechanics are also basic skills in giving sports massage.

PLANNING A SESSION

Just as the coach develops a game plan before a competition, practitioners should plan individual sports massage sessions in advance. Planning involves identifying the major goals of the session and choosing techniques and sequencing to accomplish those goals in the time allotted. The plan is usually an adaptation of a general routine or approach typically used by the massage specialist. Table 6.1 lists the elements of a session plan and general considerations for each element.

Table 6.1 Elements of Planning a Sports Massage Session

Elements	Considerations
Session goals	Type of sport
	Age
	Gender
	Current training intensity
	Today's emotional stress
	Last/next competition
	Trouble spots
	Athlete's comments
	Requests from coach, athletic trainer, others
Choosing techniques	Primary effects desired
	Secondary effects desired
Sequence of techniques	Beginning and end of session
	Effects of combination and order
	Preparing area for specific work
Routine	Time available
	Priority of session goals
	Order of massage to body regions
	Variation of routine for individuals
Environment	Adequate space
	Equipment and supplies
	Comfort of the athlete

Session Goals

Sports massage is results oriented and always has specific goals that are directly related to the athlete's performance and well-being. Examples of goals are to release tension in the neck and shoulders, to improve range of motion in the hips, to revive tired and sore feet, to relieve pain in the shins, or to de-stress after a big competition.

The goals of a particular session are determined by the immediate needs of the athlete as identified by the athlete, the coach, an athletic trainer, a health care professional, or the massage specialist. Other factors include the timing of the session in relation to an athlete's training or competition schedule and her physical, mental, and emotional condition. Each session has a general purpose depending on where it falls in the training–competition cycle, and is tailored to the individual athlete's situation.

Figure 6.1 shows the Trouble Spots Body Chart that can be used to identify and record problem areas for individual athletes. Before a session begins, ask the athlete to shade in areas of discomfort, pain, stiffness, numbness or tingling, past injury, and current injury (e.g., bruises, wounds, sprains). This chart serves as a quick visual reference and planning tool for the session.

The chart also asks for some basic information about where the athlete is in the competition cycle. When was his last event? When is his next event? How strenuous is his training right now? How far is he into the season of his sport? This information helps the practitioner identify some general session goals and create a preliminary plan of how much time to spend on certain areas or on specific outcomes.

The better the massage specialist understands the athlete and the athlete's situation, the more effective she can be in planning sessions. The answers to the following questions provide important information for massage session planning:

- What is the athlete's sport?
- Is this a pre-event, postevent, or maintenance situation?
- What are the specific problem areas to be addressed?
- Is the athlete anxious or stressed out?
- What is/are the athlete's main complaint(s)?
- Are there any complaints that need referral for diagnosis?
- Are there requests or directions from the coach, athletic trainer, other support team members?

The answers to these questions help the massage specialist prioritize goals for the session. The session plan is designed to achieve the most important goals within the time available for the massage.

Choosing Techniques

With specific goals in mind, the massage specialist chooses the appropriate massage and related techniques to use in the session. A good understanding of the primary and secondary effects of various techniques is essential in planning the best approach to achieve the session goals.

For example, to facilitate general recovery, apply deep sliding strokes, kneading, and compression to improve circulation and relax the musculature. To increase

Figure 6.1

Trouble Spots Body Chart

Name _____ Date _____

Sport _____ Age _____ Gender: **M   F**

Current training intensity (circle one):   **Easy   Moderate   High**

Today's emotional stress level (circle one):   **Low   Medium   High**

Last competition _____ Next competition _____

Please identify your body's current trouble spots on the diagram below using the trouble spots key.

KEY:
- ○ circle areas of tightness
- ● shaded circle for pain
- X "X" over stiff joints
- ≋ wavy lines over areas of numbness or tingling
- # hatch marks over recent bruises or wounds

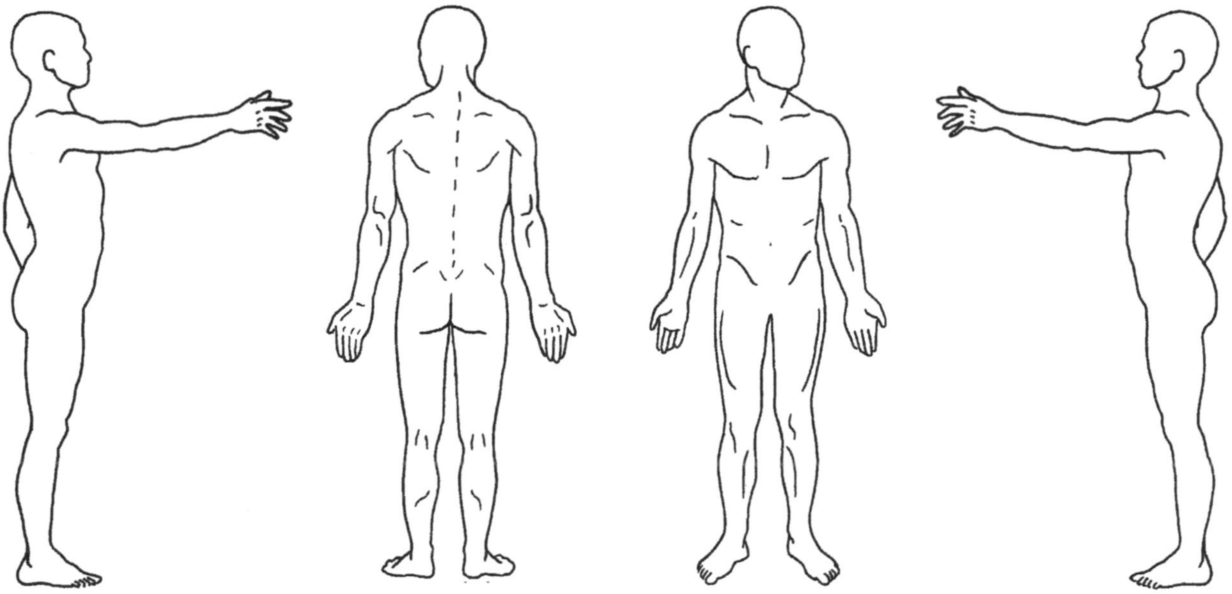

Comments _____

_____

_____

flexibility at a joint, combine deep sliding strokes and stretching. To increase pliability of muscle attachments and break adhesions, use deep transverse friction. To create a durable hyperemia in an area, perform pumping compressions. Refer to chapters 1 and 2 for more information on the effects of specific techniques.

The more experience a massage specialist has with a wide variety of techniques and technique combinations, the more successful he will be at planning and executing effective sports massage sessions (i.e., sessions that meet identified goals). Good massage specialists continually create technique variations as they work and acquire new skills through continuing education and training. They call on their entire base of knowledge and skills to achieve the session goals.

Sequence of Techniques

The sequence in which the techniques are applied can have a great effect on the outcome. A session typically begins with general techniques such as sliding strokes over a large area, then proceeds to working on a more specific area or problem, and then back to general massage to finish the session or area. The techniques used for general warm-up, specific work, connecting, and transition are listed in table 6.2.

Table 6.2 General Routine Sequence and Use of Specific Massage Techniques

General warm-up	Long sliding strokes
	Compressions
	Kneading
	Superficial skin friction
	Joint-mobilizing techniques
Specific work	Deep friction
	Vibration
	Digital compression
	Skin lifting/rolling
	Thumb slides
	Stretching
	Positional release
	Myofascial techniques
	Trigger point therapy
	Lymphatic massage
Connecting	Long sliding strokes
	Percussion
Transition	Long sliding strokes
	Joint-mobilizing techniques
Finishing	Long sliding strokes
	Percussion
	Passive touch

Sequencing may involve using one technique to prepare for or to follow up another. For example, compression and kneading may be used to prepare an area for more specific work to relieve tension in a certain muscle or muscle group, followed by stretches to help reeducate a muscle to its new length potential.

Connecting techniques are used after massage of a specific area to bring awareness back to the body as a unified whole. For example, long sliding strokes or percussion techniques to the entire leg can help reestablish a sense of wholeness after specific work on the lower leg muscles. Sliding techniques can also help create a smooth transition from one body section or subsection to another.

Finishing techniques add completeness to the session by signaling the conclusion of the massage. Massage specialists develop their own unique ways of ending a session using certain techniques, such as light sliding from head to toe, percussion, or holding the feet. They may then make a concluding statement such as, "Relax for a minute and be careful getting off of the table." The athlete then knows that the session is over.

SPORTS MASSAGE ROUTINES

No set formulas for sports massage exist—only general guidelines. However, massage specialists often develop routines or general patterns of working that they customize for each athlete receiving massage.

Massage specialists have different routines for maintenance, pre-event, inter-event, and postevent sessions. You may favor techniques that are uniquely suited to your physical capabilities or personality, and that are especially effective for you. Your routine will change as you become more experienced and learn new techniques.

Elements of a Routine

The elements of a sports massage routine are as follows:

- Order of positions
- Order of body regions
- Order of subsections

Position

The athlete's position may be supine, prone, side-lying, or sitting. A routine may include one or more positions in any order. Most sessions begin with the athlete either supine or prone. If a session is primarily focused on one area or problem, then a certain position may be preferred, such as massaging the arms with the athlete supine, or addressing the back and shoulder with the athlete prone.

Body Regions

Massage is typically performed in body regions (e.g., the head, neck, shoulder, arms, chest, abdomen, back, hips, and legs). Combinations include back and shoulders, arms and shoulders, and hips and legs. These general regions have a certain structural and functional integrity, and so it makes sense to treat them as units. However, they are also connected in many ways to the rest of the body; practitioners should keep that wholeness in mind when performing massage.

In a full-body maintenance session, a common order of addressing regions when the athlete is prone is to massage the back, the hips, and then the legs. For athletes in a supine position, the order might be legs, arms, shoulder, chest, abdomen, neck, and head. For side-lying athletes, the order might be legs, shoulder, arms, and back. For athletes in a sitting position, you might address the back, shoulder, arms, neck, and then the head. A typical order of body regions for different positions is summarized in table 6.3.

Table 6.3 Positions and Sequences of Body Regions Used in Planning a Sports Massage Routine

Position	Sequence of body regions
Prone	Back, hips, legs
Supine	Legs, arms, shoulders, chest, abdomen, neck, head
Side-lying	Legs, shoulders, arms, back
Sitting	Back, shoulders, arms, neck, head

Subsections

Subsections within different body regions are also usually massaged in a specific order. For example, after a general warm-up to the whole region, the arm is usually massaged proximal to distal (i.e., shoulder, upper arm, elbow, forearm, wrist, hand). Working in subsections increases the specificity of the massage. Table 6.4 lists a typical order for addressing subsections for the arms, legs, back, and head. Figure 6.2 shows an order of body regions for a full-body maintenance session.

The order of body regions massaged in a full-body session varies from practitioner to practitioner and becomes a signature way of working. These routines serve as a foundation for variations to address the specific needs of an athlete on a particular day.

Table 6.4 Section and Subsection Sequences Commonly Used in a Sports Massage Routine

Section	Subsection sequence
Arm	Shoulder, upper arm, elbow, forearm, wrist, hand
Leg	Hip, thigh, knee, lower leg, ankle, foot
Back	Sacroiliac, lumbar, thoracic, shoulder girdle, neck
Head	Face, jaw, scalp, neck

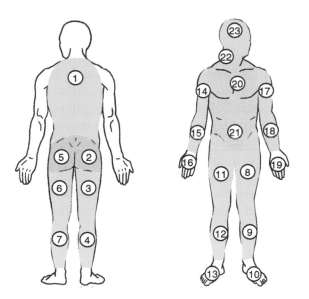

Figure 6.2 General order of body regions for full-body massage—example.

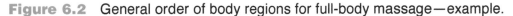

Comments on Sport-Specific Routines

Recently, some sports massage proponents have adopted the idea of creating set routines for athletes in specific sports. They reason that each sport produces its own specific stresses and strains, and so sports massage for those athletes can be prescribed. For example, a massage routine for runners is designed to focus on the lower extremities, whereas massage for racket sport players would focus on the shoulders and arms. Each sport also has its common injury sites.

Although the nature of a sport can give clues to an athlete's problem areas and injuries, the uniqueness of each athlete should not be discounted. For example, a runner who comes in with a shoulder complaint would be sorely disappointed if a massage session focused on her legs. The point of using the Trouble Spots Body Chart is to see the unique situation of the athlete who comes to you for massage.

Sports massage specialists commonly develop routine patterns of working through a session plan. However, such routines should be kept flexible, and each massage session plan should be based on the needs of the athlete, not on the sport. Set routines might be a reasonable starting point for learning sports massage, but massage specialists should quickly learn interview, assessment, and planning skills to develop individualized strategies for sports massage sessions. This approach requires both knowledge and experience, but offers better results for the individual athlete.

LOGISTICS OF GIVING SPORTS MASSAGE

In implementing the session plan, the massage specialist must create a good environment, choose the right oil or topical substance, and use good general mechanics and body mechanics. Giving sports massage also includes applying techniques with appropriate pressure, rhythm, and pacing; monitoring progress; and working in the optimal therapy zone.

Setting Up the Environment

The plan for a sports massage session should also include setting up as therapeutic an environment as possible. Sports massage may be given in a locker room, training room, or at an event site where the ideal conditions are out of the massage specialist's control. Besides having the right equipment and supplies, it is important to have enough space and, depending on the goals, relative quiet. Other factors include optimal light (not too bright or dim), optimal temperature (not too hot or cold), and a comfortable massage surface (not too hard or cold). Distractions such as other athletes talking or people walking by should be kept to a minimum. Loud, fast-paced music sometimes used during sports massage sessions should be toned down if the goal is relaxation or anxiety reduction.

HISTORY BRIEF 9

Athletic Massage c. 1940

Albert Baumgartner, a former trainer at State University of Iowa, wrote *Massage in Athletics* in 1947. One of the first books written entirely about massage for athletes, it describes classic Western massage techniques, as well as techniques developed by the German, J.B. Zabludowski (1851-1906).

According to Baumgartner, athletic massage is used for three purposes: as a *preparatory* before a workout or competition, as an *intermediate* "to maintain body energy and freshness during rest periods in practice or competition," and as *reconditioning* or recuperation after a workout to "revitalize the body."(pp. 8-9)

Baumgartner stressed the psychological effects of massage. "In the preparatory massage, for instance, the hot-headed or ardent athlete with a strong starting fever should be given only a light muscle massage of the extremities, while the phlegmatic athlete should be massaged more vigorously. . . . A good massage is half of the athlete's preparation."(p. 5)

Baumgartner also appreciated the influence of a good masseur. "The masseur, besides having technical ability, must be a good mind-reader, in order to understand the temperamental characteristics of his subjects. . . . During the massage it is easy to instill and divert courage. Upon this foregoing attribute rests the main reason for the popularity of many masseurs."(p. 101)

Baumgartner advised that "any sports trainer should be a well qualified masseur" and that "the athletic masseur should come from the ranks of professional masseurs or from the ranks of sports teachers." He admonished that "a physical education instructor should not think himself too refined to enter the profession of the athletic masseur."(p. 11)

Topical Substances

Topical substances such as oil and lotions are commonly used in sports massage, except when techniques are applied over clothing. These substances are rubbed onto the skin as lubricants to facilitate the performance of massage techniques. Botanical, homeopathic, and other ingredients are sometimes added for their therapeutic effects and to produce feelings of warmth or coolness.

Lubricants

Lubricants used in massage include oils, lotions, creams, gels, and powder. These slippery substances allow the hands to slide over the skin without irritating it and add to the smoothness of application. Massage specialists develop preferences for lubricants based on their feel (e.g., lightness or thickness), how quickly they are absorbed into the skin, ease of application and removal, and other qualities.

Vegetable oils used for massage include olive, coconut, peanut, safflower, grape seed, and almond. Oils are often mixed to achieve a certain texture and performance, and several commercial oils for sports massage are available. Massage oils are prepared differently from cooking oils, so use oil specially made for massage.

Mineral oil is also used for massage. Pure mineral oil prepared especially for massage is lightweight, does not turn rancid the way vegetable oils sometimes do, and is more easily washed out of sheets.

Lotions, *creams*, *gels*, and *powders* are other types of lubricants used for massage. Lotions, creams, and gels are less slippery than oils and are absorbed into the skin faster. They also feel less greasy and are more easily washed off. Cocoa butter prepared for use in massage is popular for deep tissue applications. Powder (e.g., powdered chalk and corn starch) is an alternative lubricant that does not leave a residue.

Active Healing Ingredients

Botanical and homeopathic substances are sometimes added to base substances for their healing effects on minor injuries such as bruises, strains, sprains, and inflammation. These active healing ingredients are found in many of the commercial preparations sold for massage.

Essential oils are concentrated essences of aromatic plants that have healing properties. They are used in small quantities and mixed with base oils for certain therapeutic effects. Essential oils useful for their calming effects include lavender, clary sage, sandalwood, and chamomile. Eucalyptus, rosemary, peppermint, and lemon are used for stimulation and mental clarity. Juniper enhances a sense of strength and well-being and is thought to ease muscle and joint pain. Arnica also eases pain from bruises and muscle strain. *Homeopathic ingredients* are sometimes mixed with essential oils in special preparations.

Warmth and Coolness

Topical substances that produce warmth or coolness are popular among athletes. Although they should be used sparingly during massage, they can be applied near the end of the session for their "feel good" effects. The practitioner should ask for the athlete's permission to use these products since people have differing reactions to them.

Rubefacients are popular for minor muscle soreness and stiff joints. The active ingredients in rubefacients are camphor and eucalyptus, or in herbal preparations are black pepper, juniper, and rosemary. These substances increase local superficial circulation by causing mild irritation of the skin and produce a reddening (rube) and warming effect. Rubefacients come in watery concoctions called liniments, and in gels and creams in familiar brand names such as Ben-Gay and Tiger Balm. The warmth produced feels good, but their actual therapeutic effects are superficial.

Substances that have a cooling effect on the skin are preferred by some athletes to relieve sore muscles and joints and arthritis pain. These cryo-substances come in creams, gels, and liniments. The active ingredients include menthol, camphor, and peppermint.

Astringents such as witch hazel and rubbing alcohol also feel cool on the skin and are applied for stimulation and to close pores. They are watery and can be used to remove oil from the athlete's skin after massage.

Cautions

Always check with athletes to make sure that they are not allergic to the topical substance you plan to use, and that it will not irritate their skin. Many of the preparations marketed for sports massage are strong smelling and can irritate the skin, even causing burning if rubbed in too forcefully. Apply substances with strong ingredients such as camphor and menthol after massage of an area as a finishing move.

Ingredients that cause warming or cooling of the skin should not be used with hot packs or cold therapies. Avoid mixing preparations that may interact negatively or multiply an effect (e.g., warming) to a dangerous level.

General Mechanics

General mechanics refers to positioning the client, handling pillows and bolsters, draping properly, and using towels and sheets. These are practical aspects of giving massage beyond the application of techniques.

Athletes may lie supine, prone, or in a side-lying position on a massage table, or they may be seated in a special massage chair. Figures 6.3 to 6.6 show these common positions for massage. Pillows and bolsters are used to position athletes comfortably and to relieve stress on certain areas. For example, for athletes lying supine, bolsters are placed under the knees and neck. For athletes in the prone position, bolsters are placed under the ankles and shoulders, and the face cradle is adjusted for good neck alignment (see figure 6.4). For side-lying athletes, bolsters go under the head, upper arm, and upper leg (see figure 6.5).

Bolsters may be moved according to what you are trying to accomplish. For example, in the side-lying position a bolster is typically placed under the top knee for support and to keep the hip in a neutral position. However, the bolster is removed when the intention is to work the IT (or ilio-tibial band) in a stretched position, or to place the gluteus and piriformis muscles in a stretch.

When the athlete is changing position (e.g., from prone to supine or from supine to side-lying), you should hold and adjust the drape. You should also guide the athlete through the movement to minimize awkwardness and "undoing" the effects of the massage.

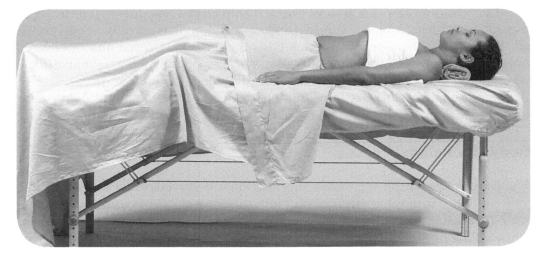

Figure 6.3   Use of bolsters for support and proper draping for a female athlete in supine position.

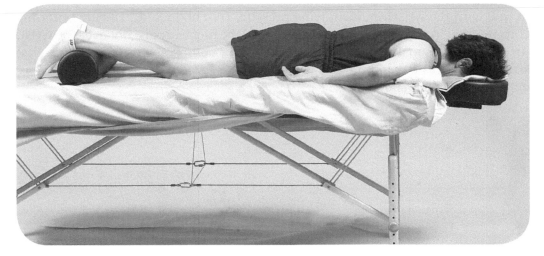

Figure 6.4   Use of bolsters for support in the prone position.

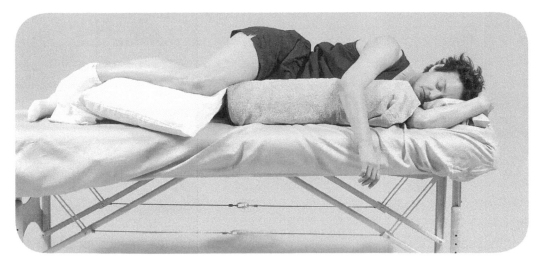

Figure 6.5   Use of bolsters for support in the side-lying position.

Proper draping allows you to work unencumbered while preserving the modesty of the athlete. Athletes' genitals and women's breasts should be covered at all times with a sheet or towel. Each body region is uncovered and re-covered as the session progresses. Figure 6.3 shows proper draping for a woman athlete when massaging the muscles on the chest, shoulders, or abdomen.

Sheets and towels are used for draping and when applying hot or cold packs. Rolled towels are useful as small bolsters.

Body Mechanics

The *body mechanics* of the massage practitioner deserve special attention. Just as an athlete can develop physical problems because of poor posture and biomechanics, massage practitioners can damage their bodies by the way they use them while giving massage. The most common injuries involve the thumb and wrists, tendinitis from repetitive motion, and chronic tension in the back and neck.

Principles of good body mechanics include keeping the back in alignment and the head over the shoulders, bending at the knees to lower the body, keeping wrists in a neutral position (not flexed or extended), and keeping thumbs in line with the wrist when applying pressure (not abducted). During pumping compression, reinforce the bottom hand over the metacarpals, not over the wrist. An alternative is to use the back of a loose fist for compressions to keep the wrist straight. Figures 6.6 and 6.7 show good posture for giving massage. (For more details, see Dixon, 2001.)

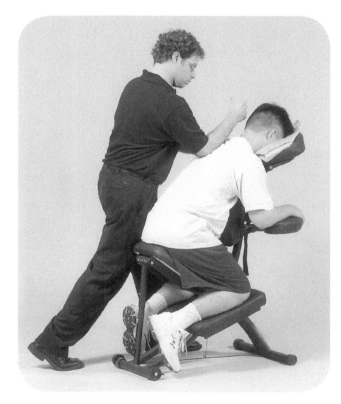

Figure 6.6 Positioning for massage in a special massage chair.

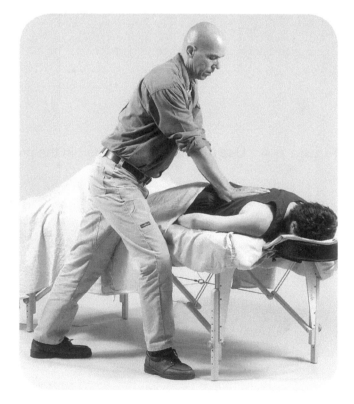

Figure 6.7 Good body mechanics for giving massage.

ASPECTS OF TECHNIQUE PERFORMANCE

The most important aspects of massage technique performance are pressure, rhythm, pacing, continuity, and specificity. Variations in these qualities determine the physical, mental, and emotional effects produced. Table 6.5 lists the important aspects of massage performance and the range of their variations.

Table 6.5   **Important Aspects of Massage Technique Performance**

Performance aspect	Variations
Pressure	Light to moderate to heavy
Rhythm	Even or uneven
Pacing	Slow to moderate to fast
Continuity	Smooth or choppy transitions
Specificity	General area to specific structure
	General goal to specific intent

Pressure

The pressure used in applying a technique should be appropriate for the type and condition of the tissue and the body part receiving massage. Pressure may vary from light on sensitive areas; to moderate on normal tissues; to heavy on healthy, heavily muscled areas. Working on a sore area with heavy pressure might cause tissue damage or protective spasm and should be avoided. Working too lightly will not have the desired effect. Further discussion of finding the right pressure for remedial and rehabilitation applications can be found in the upcoming section on the optimal therapy zone.

During a session, a body region is warmed up and prepared using light pressure at first, and then gradually deepening pressure as massage of the area progresses. This allows the athlete receiving massage to adapt to the touch of the practitioner and prepares the tissues for more vigorous movement—much like a warm-up in sports.

Rhythm, Pacing, and Continuity

The rhythm and pacing of the massage application are important to establish continuity and flow and effect either relaxation or stimulation. For example, fast-paced percussion is stimulating, whereas slower kneading and sliding strokes are more relaxing.

Smooth transitions from one technique to another add a sense of continuity. Once contact is made with the athlete, it should not be broken abruptly. Skillful transitions from one body region to another contribute to a feeling of continuity and depend on good draping skills.

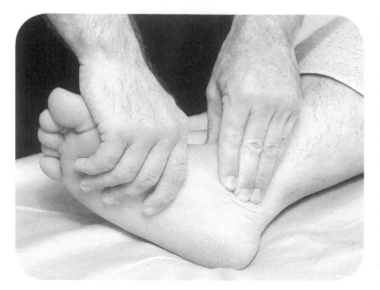

Figure 6.8 Specificity in applying friction to the ankle ligaments.

Specificity

Specificity refers to the size of the area being massaged, whether the effects are general or local, and the focus on a particular structure (e.g., a specific muscle or tendon). The smaller the area, the more local the effects, and the more defined the structure, the more you are said to be working with specificity.

Some techniques such as palmar compression affect a wide area and so are considered less specific. Techniques such as deep transverse friction on a tendon and thumb pressure to a trigger point affect very small areas and are considered more specific. Figure 6.8 shows specific work on the ankle ligaments.

The ability to work with specificity comes with knowledge and experience. It is the product of knowing the location of anatomical structures, being able to palpate small structures or subtle differences in tissues, and being skilled in certain massage techniques.

MONITORING PROGRESS AND PAIN

During a massage session, you get feedback from the athlete in a number of ways. You get information from palpation and your own sense of touch, from the athlete's comments and answers to your questions, and also from the athlete's reaction to any pain felt as you apply techniques.

Monitoring pain can be one of the most valuable methods of feedback. Pain is especially important for safety because it may be an indication of damage to the tissues and signal a contraindication for certain techniques or movements. Athletes can learn to distinguish between "good pain" and "bad pain" much as they do when working out or performing.

People have different tolerances for pain and varying emotional responses to it. Some brace or tighten their muscles against pain, which, although natural, is counterproductive during massage. Some are stoic and give no apparent feedback either verbally or with facial expressions or body language. These athletes may sustain damage to tissues before they acknowledge any pain.

Some theories of massage recommend avoiding pain altogether. This is true for massage at events and for general recovery. However, for remedial and rehabilitation situations, pain may offer a signal that a therapeutic benefit is taking place. The optimal therapy zone theory, discussed in the following section, describes how to monitor pain in the latter situation.

Optimal Therapy Zone

The concept of the *optimal therapy zone (OTZ)* is very useful in remedial and rehabilitation applications of massage (Lamp, 1989). The OTZ is best described as the amount of pressure (depth) needed to have a therapeutic effect.

The OTZ is typically found when the pressure is enough to cause some discomfort, but not enough to cause voluntary or involuntary splinting of the muscles in the area. The practitioner must remain sensitive to the amount of pain the athlete is experiencing and avoid causing too much in an effort to get quick results. Achieving the OTZ is like trying to erase a mistake on a piece of paper—not enough pressure and it will not erase; too much pressure and the paper tears.

Working in the OTZ is effective when the goal of the session is one of the following:

- Releasing chronic muscle hypertonicity
- Helping the athlete form healthy scar tissue
- Healing tendinitis
- Breaking up adhesions
- Deactivating trigger points
- Increasing range of motion
- Healing subclinical muscle–tendon problems
- Preventing problems resulting from biomechanical stress

Each situation has its own OTZ. The OTZ is not defined by a set amount of pressure; rather, it is determined by several factors related to the body part being massaged, the nature of the condition or injury, and the tolerance of the athlete.

Some areas of the body are more sensitive than others. For example, the presence of adipose tissue seems to decrease pain tolerance and increase the chance of delayed-onset muscle soreness after a massage session. Adipose tissue also bruises more easily than lean tissue.

An athlete in good condition will typically have a higher pain tolerance than the norm for the general population. The more extensive the injury, the lower the pain tolerance will be. If the athlete is sick with a cold or the flu, depressed, or worried, pain tolerance seems to decrease. The level of confidence in the practitioner also seems to have an effect on an athlete's pain tolerance. When athletes are unsure of massage specialists' skills, or doubtful of their sympathy, the level of apprehension rises while pain tolerance tends to drop. Finally, the athlete's need or desire to recover quickly can result in higher pain tolerance. For example, if an athlete's livelihood is his sport, or if his self-esteem or peer acceptance is at stake, he may better tolerate the pain of rehabilitation.

The optimal therapy zone also includes using appropriate techniques for the situation. Working in the OTZ often involves such techniques as deep transverse friction, deep digital pressure, deep thumb slides, and broadening.

Treatment within the OTZ should be 10 minutes or less, sometimes as short as 30 seconds. The practitioner should move in and out of the OTZ and alternate techniques to give some relief from the discomfort of working in the zone. If the athlete's pain tolerance begins to decrease significantly, treatment in the OTZ should be discontinued for that session.

Sports massage specialists performing massage for rehabilitation should be knowledgeable about working with injuries and ice modalities, and skillful in deep massage techniques. They should have good communication skills in both talking and listening, and be empathetic and supportive.

A "ruthless compassion" is needed to encourage the athlete to accept the treatment in the face of pain. Practitioners should be aggressive, but not overzealous. They should be in control, but allow the athlete to have the final word about when enough is enough.

The day after working in the OTZ, the athlete may experience some soreness. However, she should not feel severe soreness or have bruising. This would indicate that too much pressure was used. Delayed-onset soreness can be minimized by icing the area after the treatment. Practitioners who check in with athletes the day after treatment in the OTZ can get feedback about their degree of success.

Why work in the OTZ if it causes pain? Because it gives faster results, a quicker return to optimal function, and less time away from training.

Now you have the basics of why, when, and how to give an effective sports massage. Chapter 7 presents the nuts and bolts of implementing a sports massage program for a school, club, or team, or at an individual sport event.

STUDY QUESTIONS

1. What does it mean that sports massage is results oriented?
2. How is the Trouble Spots Body Chart used to determine session goals?
3. What are three important questions to ask in identifying session goals?
4. Which massage techniques are used for each of the following: warm-up, specific work, connecting, transitioning, and finishing a session?
5. If the athlete is supine on the massage table, in what order would you address different body regions? What about athletes who are prone, side-lying, and sitting?
6. In what order would you massage the subsections of an athlete's arm? What about the leg, back, and head?
7. Why should sports massage *not* be based on prescribed sport-specific routines?
8. What are important considerations in setting up the environment for sports massage?
9. What are the choices for lubricants used in sports massage?
10. How do different active ingredients enhance a sports massage session?
11. What are the cautions in using topical substances in sports massage?
12. How do you determine how much pressure to use in performing massage?
13. How do you vary the rhythm and pacing of massage for different effects?
14. What gives a massage application specificity? Why is that an important quality?
15. Where do you place bolsters when positioning an athlete lying supine on a massage table? What about an athlete lying prone and side-lying?
16. What are the important aspects of body mechanics when giving massage?
17. In what ways can massage specialists damage their hands when giving massage?
18. How is pain used to monitor progress during massage?
19. What is the optimal therapy zone? When do you work in the OTZ?
20. What are some important safety considerations when working in the OTZ?

CHAPTER 7

IMPLEMENTING A SPORTS MASSAGE PROGRAM

LEARNING OUTCOMES

1. Identify ways to procure a massage specialist for a school program.
2. Plan a schedule for sports massage for a season.
3. Describe how athletes and coaches can be part of a sports massage program.
4. Explain the concentric circle model of the athlete's support team.
5. Explain how athletic organizations use sports massage.
6. Outline general guidelines for sports massage teams at events.
7. Describe how sports massage is offered at health clubs.
8. Describe a private sports massage practice.
9. Explain the role of the massage specialist in a sports medicine clinic.

SPORTS MASSAGE PROGRAMS

You are convinced of the value of sports massage for enhancing the health and performance of athletes. Now you must decide how to implement a sports massage program. How do you find and fund a sports massage specialist? Where do you find the space and time? Who gets massage? How often? For what purpose? How do sports massage specialists interact with coaches, athletic trainers, and physicians?

School and university athletic departments, amateur and professional athletic organizations, organized athletic events, health clubs, private massage practices, and integrative sports medicine clinics all provide sports massage services. Each setting has a unique set of circumstances to consider when implementing its program. This chapter considers sports massage programs in a variety of settings and the role of the massage specialist on the athlete's support team.

SCHOOL AND UNIVERSITY PROGRAMS

Some school and university athletic departments use the full range of possibilities for sports massage: event, maintenance, and rehabilitation. Others provide one aspect or another (e.g., only recovery massage after practices, regular maintenance, or only event sports massage). However extensive the sports massage program, certain questions need to be answered regarding how to find and fund a massage specialist; what space, equipment, and supplies to provide; how to schedule sessions; and how to involve coaches, assistants, and athletes themselves in using massage in the sport setting.

Finding and Funding a Massage Specialist

How do you find a qualified sports massage specialist? Look for graduates of massage training programs that include sports massage as a specialty, or locate a massage therapist who has had continuing education in sports massage. Some massage schools and professional associations for massage therapists have teams that provide pre-event and postevent massage for amateur competitions. Professional associations also have lists of massage therapists who specialize in sports massage. Contact the American Massage Therapy Association at www.amtamassage.org or the Associated Bodywork and Massage Professionals organization at www.abmp.com.

Your state or local government may require a license to practice massage, although some laws exempt those working with athletic teams. Appendix B lists the contact information for state licensing authorities. Be sure that any massage specialist you hire has a valid license if one is required by law.

Massage specialists should also carry professional liability insurance. Many obtain their insurance as professional members of an association.

In school and university athletic programs with tight budgets, funding a massage specialist can be a challenge. Funds may come from the regular athletic budget or from outside sources. In some cases, a booster club for a school or specific team provides the funds for a sports massage program.

Massage in Physical Education and Athletics

Swedish immigrants and Americans who had studied at the Royal Central Institute in Stockholm brought P.H. Ling's educational and medical gymnastics to the United States in the 1850s. Ling's systems of active and passive exercise were to gain popularity in school physical education programs and as the Swedish Movement Cure.

Dio Lewis' Normal Institute of Physical Culture offered instruction in Ling's systems as early as 1862. Hartvig Nissen, Sweden's vice-consul to the United States, opened the Swedish Health Institute for the Treatment of Chronic Diseases by Swedish Movements and Massage in Washington, D.C., in 1893. Baron Nils Posse opened the Normal School of Physical Education that also maintained clinics in several Boston hospitals in the 1890s. Graduates of Posse's program were trained in both educational and medical gymnastics, modeling Ling's school in Stockholm.

Many of the reconstruction aides who used massage, Swedish movements, and hydrotherapy to rehabilitate soldiers wounded in World War I were trained in schools of physical education. In 1928 Stafford wrote, "The branches of physiotherapy which have been and will continue to be handled by physical educators are those of massage and therapeutic exercise and certain phases of heat and water treatments."(p. xiii)

This tradition continued into the 1950s with physical education programs serving as training grounds for future physical therapists. This connection to physiotherapy is evident in today's athletic training and in a small number of kinesiotherapy programs still offered in physical education departments.

In physical education and athletic departments, the ancient tradition of massage for athletes passed down informally through generations of trainers was enriched by developments in massage and physiotherapy in the early 1900s. In 1915, R. Tait McKenzie spoke of the benefits of athletic massage as common knowledge among trainers.

> Its action in improving muscle tone, in postponing the onset of fatigue and hastening recovery from it, has long been recognized by athletic trainers. In preparing athletes for a contest, general massage is always given by friction, kneading, pinching, and stroking, lubricating the surface with some oily liniment. After a hard race or other contest it is a matter of common knowledge among trainers that a five-minute [massage] treatment will enable an athlete to repeat or continue a performance otherwise impossible. (p. 340)

Given its heritage, sports massage naturally is again finding a welcome place among athletes and school athletic departments across North America.

Massage specialists often work on contract and are usually paid by the hour or by the session. They may also be employees of a school or athletic organization, similar to athletic trainers. Responsible students can be trained as assistant massage specialists, much like student trainers. They might work under the supervision of a massage specialist, coach, or trainer.

Just as the athletic trainer should be available to all, in an ideal situation, a sports massage program should serve all student athletes. To accomplish this, school programs can hire several sports massage specialists, train student assistants, teach self-massage and partner massage, or do some combination. Student interns from a local massage school are another potential resource. With a firm commitment, good planning, and a little creativity, school athletic program coordinators can find resources for a sports massage program.

Space, Equipment, and Supplies

Ideally, a special room for massage is set aside, but space can be improvised in a training room, locker room, or office. Massage specialists may travel with a team to important competitive events and set up a massage room at the hotel where athletes are staying. At individual sport competitions, spaces are often set aside for massage by event organizers. Check with event planners in advance to see if they have provided a suitable space for massage.

Massage specialists often have their own equipment, but the school may want to provide a portable massage table or massage chair for use at home and away events. A tent or other shelter is often used at outdoor events to shield practitioners and athletes from the sun and rain.

Supplies include massage oils and other topical substances, paper towels, alcohol solution spray bottles, and perhaps an electric vibration device. Sheets and towels may be needed for draping depending on the type of massage offered. Massage specialists sometimes have their own small hand tools (e.g., T-bars) for applying specific pressure to points. Heating packs and ice should be available for use as adjunct therapies.

Master Schedule

A master schedule for sports massage with a particular team is useful in order to see the big picture of its place in a program over a period of time such as a specific competitive season. Ideally, a master schedule for sports massage is developed by the team of sport professionals including the coach, athletic trainer, athletic department, and sports massage specialist. The master schedule will be altered as the season progresses and other schedules shift, athletes develop certain needs, competitions are added or deleted, and other factors change.

Developing a master schedule of sports massage sessions requires taking into consideration practice and nonpractice days, time available before and after practices, and time around competitions. Other factors to consider include duration (e.g., 30 or 60 minutes), frequency of sessions (e.g., times per week), and space availability.

A session's duration depends on its proximity to competition, the time available overall, the number of athletes involved, and the objectives to be accomplished. The time will vary with different situations. Blocks of time can be set aside for sports massage, and the sessions within that block can be planned on the actual day of the sessions according to the athletes' needs.

Scheduling massage for team sports presents more of a challenge than for individual sports. For example, in sports such as basketball, football, field hockey, and soccer, players warm up as a team, whereas the pre-event preparation for individual sports is more solitary. Pre-event massage for a whole team might not make much sense; however, individual athletes on a team may benefit from a quick pregame massage. Recovery and maintenance massage can be scheduled over a longer period of time and can be given regularly after and between games.

Instructing athletes in self-massage and partner massage might also be part of a master plan. Coaches may want to be trained themselves in how to massage their athletes. Figure 7.1 shows a sample master schedule for sports massage for a track team in a one-month period.

Sports Massage by Athletes and Coaches

Athletes can learn to do self-massage and partner massage for a variety of situations including warm-ups, preactivity and postactivity, and general recovery. Experienced sports massage specialists can teach simple and effective no-oil massage techniques in a workshop. With some follow-up supervision, this should be sufficient to start athletes giving massage to themselves and each other. (Refer to King, 1993, for layman's information on no-oil sports massage techniques.)

Sunday	Monday	Tuesday	Wednesday	Thursday	Friday	Saturday
Rest day	Practice	Practice SMS*—1/2 hour maintenance sessions	Practice Workshop on partner and self-massage	Practice	Travel Short practice SMS—1/2 hour sessions in preparation for meet	All-day meet SMS—pre-, inter-, and postevent sessions
Rest day	Practice	Practice SMS—1/2 hour maintenance sessions	Practice	Local meet SMS—pre-, inter-, and postevent sessions	Short practice SMS—1/2 hour recovery sessions	Practice
Rest day	Practice	Practice SMS—1/2 hour maintenance sessions	Practice	Practice	Travel Short practice SMS—1/2 hour sessions in preparation for meet	Weekend meet SMS—pre-, inter-, and postevent sessions
Weekend meet SMS—pre-, inter-, and postevent sessions	Short practice	Practice SMS—1/2 hour maintenance sessions	Practice	Practice	Practice	Local meet SMS—pre-, inter-, and postevent sessions

*SMS = Sports massage specialist

Figure 7.1 Master schedule for sports massage for a track team for one month of a competitive season.

In addition, coaches may want their own training to learn how they can use massage to enhance their coaching. Because of their special relationship to athletes, coaches might use massage differently—for example, when giving last-minute instructions before a performance or for psychological effects.

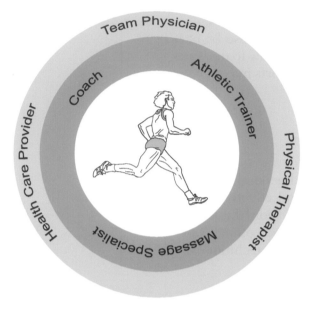

Figure 7.2 The athlete's support team— concentric circle model.

THE ATHLETE'S SUPPORT TEAM

What is the place of the sports massage specialist in relation to other members of the athlete's support team? Traditionally, sports massage specialists have a broad range of functions from health maintenance, to preparation for events and recovery afterwards, to remedial and rehabilitation applications. Ideally the sports massage specialist is a part of the athlete's total support network, which includes the other professionals who care for the athletes.

A good comprehensive model for the athlete's support team is the concentric circle model. This model includes an inner circle and an outer circle (see figure 7.2). The inner circle represents professionals who focus on enhancing performance, and the outer circle represents those who treat injuries. All members of the support team work in dynamic relationship to each other.

Inner Circle of the Support Team

The innermost circle of the athlete's support team consists of those concerned specifically with performance enhancement, injury prevention, and addressing minor injuries and complaints. These are the coaches, athletic trainers, and massage specialists.

Years ago, a single person called the trainer performed all three inner circle functions. Since the 1950s, specializations have emerged for different parts of the trainer's role. Athletes now rely on a team of trainers, each focusing on a particular aspect of preparing them for top sport performance. Given this common history, it is not surprising to see some overlap in the training and functions of coaches, athletic trainers, and massage specialists.

Generally speaking, coaches are responsible for developing the athlete's sport skills and overseeing their sport performance and physical conditioning. Athletic trainers assess, treat, and rehabilitate injuries. Sports massage specialists focus on recovery, physical and mental preparation for competition, and minor problem conditions. All are concerned with injury prevention.

Massage has traditionally been used to prepare athletes for the physical exertion of training sessions and competitions and for recovery afterwards. These aspects of sports massage are concerned with the healthy athlete and the enhancement of normal physical and mental functioning.

As mentioned previously, the experienced massage specialist can often detect abnormalities in tissues, joint movement, and mental and emotional states before they lead to performance deterioration or to debilitating pain and dysfunction. The massage specialist can alert the coach or athletic trainer to potential problem conditions so they can assess the situation themselves and modify the athlete's training accordingly.

Maintenance massage can address problem areas and restore conditions to a more normal state before they become chronic problems or acute injuries. Massage specialists also address minor complaints and injuries, such as tight and sore muscles, and refer athletes with more serious conditions to the athletic trainer.

The athletic trainer typically evaluates complaints, gives first aid, and does preventative taping to minimize the chance of injury or reinjury and for rehabilitation. The athletic trainer might refer athletes to the massage specialist in cases in which massage would be beneficial.

Outer Circle of the Support Team

When an athlete's condition or complaint requires further care or diagnosis, the case moves to the outer circle of the support team. The intermediary for the referral is most often the athletic trainer. Typically the coach and the massage specialist refer problem conditions and complaints to the athletic trainer. The athletic trainer, in turn, refers athletes to the team physician or other appropriate health care provider.

Once the condition is diagnosed and a rehabilitation program is planned, the athlete may receive rehabilitation from a sport physical therapist, or may return to the inner circle of the support team for treatment from the athletic trainer or massage specialist. The athletic trainer is usually the coordinator for rehabilitation and is in contact with the team physician.

The involvement of massage specialists in rehabilitation varies with the situation and with their training in medical or clinical massage and in treating musculoskeletal injuries. Massage facilitates soft tissue healing and the formation of healthy scar tissue and can help keep the rest of the body healthy while the injury is healing. Massage can also have psychological benefits related to reducing anxiety and increasing feelings of well-being for athletes sidelined by injuries.

To use their skills fully, massage specialists must interact with coaches and athletic trainers on a regular and ongoing basis. In a comprehensive program, athletes would also receive maintenance sports massage regularly (at least weekly or biweekly) and before and after competitions. Massage specialists would be familiar with the athletes; their sports; and their physical, mental, and emotional states. They would see athletes regularly enough to note significant changes and tailor their sessions to the athletes' immediate and long-term needs.

ATHLETIC ORGANIZATIONS

Many professional and amateur athletes hire their own massage specialists. This is a common practice in individual sports such as running, tennis, figure skating, boxing, and cycling, sports in which athletes have their own coaches, athletic trainers, personal physicians, and other support staff. Sometimes tournament managers (e.g., on a professional tennis circuit) provide a massage specialist for all players. An Olympic team may have its own massage specialist who travels with the team to training camp and to the Games themselves.

Some professional sport teams hire team massage therapists to provide massage to all team members. This assures that athletes will at least receive regular postevent massage, maintenance massage, or both. The logistics of providing massage in those circumstances is similar to in schools (i.e., creating a master schedule, allocating space, providing equipment, and making travel arrangements).

ORGANIZED SPORT EVENTS

One of most publicly recognized settings for sports massage today is organized athletic events. Teams of sports massage specialists are visible at such prestigious events as the Olympic Games, Pan-American Games, Goodwill Games, and international marathons such as the Boston Marathon. They are also found at regional and local fund-raising runs and walks and at school track and swim meets.

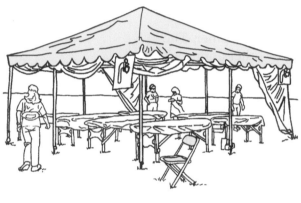

A sports massage team is typically composed of several massage specialists who provide massage to competitors at the event. Figure 7.3 shows a shelter setup for sports massage at an outdoor event. Event organizers view sports massage as either a separate service for athletes or a part of a medical team. Corporate sponsors may fund sports massage teams.

Sports massage at organized events differs from sports massage in other settings because here a specialist is most often working on strangers and for a limited period of time—sometimes as little as 15 minutes each. Postevent massage might also involve first aid and recognizing the signs of more serious conditions and injuries that should be referred to the medical team. Postevent massage should be well coordinated.

Figure 7.3 Sports massage at an outdoor event.

General Guidelines for Sports Massage Teams

Following are some general guidelines for organizing a sports massage team for an event.

☐ Establish criteria for sports massage team members (e.g., training, experience, license).

☐ Recruit qualified massage practitioners well in advance of the event.

☐ Arrange for funding via a general event budget or corporate sponsorship.

☐ Get agreements in writing and be sure they are signed by the proper authorities.

☐ Clearly define the scope of responsibility for the sports massage team and its relationship to other event staff members, especially the medical team.

☐ Meet with event organizers to review the logistics of providing sports massage (e.g., how many athletes are expected, how many massage sessions will be given, provisions for a shelter, who provides and pays for supplies, identification badges and other security measures, and "freebies" such as T-shirts for massage volunteers).

☐ Organize the event massage operation (e.g., traffic flow in the massage area, arrangement of tables, athlete sign-up with release forms, assignment of athletes to tables, use of assistants).

☐ Arrange for an orientation of massage specialists close to the event time to go over logistics, the protocol for referral to the medical team, and last-minute instructions.

☐ Address other concerns (e.g., parking, breaks, snacks, timing the sessions).

Supplies

Supplies may be provided by the event organization or corporate sponsor. Some may be brought by massage specialists themselves. Supplies for sports massage at events include the following:

☐ Plastic fitted sheets to protect massage tables

☐ Alcohol solution to sanitize the table or a plastic sheet between athletes

☐ Paper towels to wipe tables and clean hands between sessions

☐ A garbage bag for paper towels

☐ Blankets, space blankets, and head and hand coverings for first aid for athletes with hypothermia

☐ Water for fluid replacement and warm broth in cold weather

☐ Ice, baggies, and ice cups for first aid

☐ Bleach solution (1 part bleach to 10 parts water) or other disinfectant, and latex gloves (See appendix A for situations in which blood or other body fluids are present.)

☐ Sunscreen, a hat, bug spray, and snacks for massage specialists

☐ Miscellaneous useful items such as spray bottles, cotton towels, masking tape, and a clipboard and paper for signing in athletes

Coordinating With the Medical Team

Ideally, a sports massage team at an organized event such as a marathon or fundraising walk coordinates its efforts with the event's medical team. Following are some suggestions for event organizers:

○ Develop a protocol for referral of injured athletes from the massage area to the medical area.

○ Establish a clear path for movement between the massage and medical areas.

○ Station someone from the medical team in the sports massage area to handle emergencies (e.g., an emergency medical technician [EMT]).

○ Station some experienced massage specialists in the medical area to help with situations in which massage might be beneficial (e.g., muscle cramp relief).

HEALTH CLUBS

Most health clubs offer massage to their members, and they may need a massage establishment license to offer this service. Scheduling and paying for massage in this setting is the athlete's personal responsibility. The massage program manager makes sure that massage practitioners are available at popular times such as after classes and during local competitions.

Well-run health clubs educate their members about the benefits of massage. Marketing massage services might include flyers, bulletin board displays, lectures, and short announcements during activity classes. The more knowledgeable about massage other staff persons (e.g., personal trainers, teachers, desk personnel) are, the more likely they will be to recommend it to club members.

The sports massage specialist may confer with activity instructors and personal trainers to better serve mutual clients. A massage specialist may, with further training, double as a personal trainer.

When setting up a massage program at a health club, locate the massage room in an area with easy access to locker rooms. This makes dressing easier and offers better access to showers, steam rooms, saunas, whirlpools, and other locker room facilities. Also try to find a relatively quiet location. A room near or below an aerobics studio or next to the racquetball courts or weight room might be too noisy for relaxing massage.

If a number of massage specialists are involved, a massage program coordinator or manager can plan schedules, keep records, and take care of other administrative details. Massage practitioners at health clubs work as independent contractors or employees depending on the circumstances. Managers should check IRS rules for independent contractors and employees to be sure they are following applicable guidelines.

PRIVATE SPORTS MASSAGE PRACTICES

Many sports massage specialists maintain private practices in their own offices and clinics. Athletes seeking massage specialists are taking personal responsibility for their own health care, and they make the effort to contact the specialist and to schedule and pay for their sessions.

Sports massage specialists work with their athlete clients to schedule regular maintenance sessions, special preparatory sessions before big events, and recovery sessions afterwards. Minor remedial conditions are addressed during maintenance sessions.

Much like those working in health clubs, sports massage specialists in private practice have to educate potential athlete clients and advertise their services. Working on sports massage teams for organized events or giving talks at local sports clubs are excellent ways to meet potential clients.

In the absence of ready-made sports medicine programs such as in the school team setting, individual sports massage specialists develop their own systems for referrals and communication with coaches, personal trainers, physicians, chiropractors, and other health care professionals who work with athletes.

INTEGRATIVE SPORTS MEDICINE CLINICS

Integrative sports medicine clinics specialize in the rehabilitation of athletes suffering from sport- and activity-related injuries, as well as in improving athletic performance. These clinics are essentially medical settings with a specialization in athletes. Clinic staff typically includes physical therapists, athletic trainers, and massage therapists. Medical staff might include orthopedic doctors, physiatrists (i.e., doctors specializing in musculoskeletal conditions), chiropractors, or other primary health care providers who focus on the needs of athletes.

People go to sports medicine clinics because they want health care providers who understand their needs as athletes. They are physically active and want to continue to be active as much as possible while healing from injuries. Athletes also want to go beyond a normal functional level (ADL, or activities of daily living) to a physical condition that enhances their sport performance. Rehabilitation for athletes includes strengthening and flexibility exercises that help them meet their performance goals.

Massage specialists in integrative sports medicine clinics provide massage for all the usual reasons (e.g., improve tissue health, increase circulation, relaxation). But because athletes go to sports medicine clinics with injuries and some level of dysfunction, these massage specialists must also be experts in soft tissue injuries. They work closely with other health care professionals in planning and executing treatment and rehabilitation plans.

STUDY QUESTIONS

1. How do you find a qualified sports massage specialist?
2. What are space, equipment, and supplies requirements for offering sports massage in different settings?
3. What are the important considerations in planning a master schedule for sports massage during a competitive season?
4. How can athletes, assistants, and coaches contribute to a sports massage program?
5. In what ways do athletic organizations and teams provide sports massage?
6. What are the general guidelines for organizing a sports massage team?
7. What are essential supplies for sports massage at events?
8. How are the sports massage team and medical team coordinated at events?
9. In what ways does the setup for sports massage at health clubs differ from that provided in school athletic programs?
10. How does the role of the sports massage specialist in school programs differ from their role in private sports massage practices?
11. What is the role of the sports massage specialist in an integrative sports medicine clinic?

SANITARY GUIDELINES FOR SPORTS MASSAGE AT EVENTS

The following sanitary guidelines, sometimes called universal precautions, are intended to prevent the transmission of serious communicable diseases such as HIV, hepatitis B, and other blood-borne pathogens. Although sports massage specialists are generally at low risk for contact with blood-borne pathogens, the probability of coming into contact with blood increases while working at sports events. Chafing, blood blisters on the feet, and road rash from falls are all common occurrences at road races, triathlons, and bicycle events.

1. Use protective barriers, such as latex gloves, to prevent contact with blood, body fluids containing visible blood, or other body fluids to which universal precautions apply.* When removing gloves, take them off inside out; wash hands with bleach solution or other appropriate disinfectant.

2. If you come into contact with blood or other body fluids that can transmit disease, use these precautions:
   a. Wash hands with a bleach solution of 1 part bleach to 10 parts water.
   b. Immediately and thoroughly wash the table and other surfaces that have had contact with the fluid.
   c. Put all waste materials (e.g., paper towels) into a separate plastic bag. This may be considered medical waste, and it should be disposed of properly. Check with medical personnel at the event site for proper protocol.

3. Take care to prevent injuries when using sharp instruments or, more common for sports massage specialists, when in the medical area where sharp instruments (e.g., needles) are being used.

For more information, see U.S. Department of Health and Human Services, Centers for Disease Control and Prevention (CDC) at www.cdc.gov.

*Universal precautions also apply to certain body fluids with which massage specialists are not likely to come in contact (i.e., blood, semen and vaginal/cervical secretions, urine, feces, and vomit). Universal precautions do not apply to the following fluids, unless they contain visible blood, because the risk of transmission of disease is extremely low or nonexistent: nasal secretions, saliva, sweat, tears, sputum.

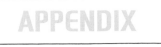
MASSAGE LICENSING LAWS

The following list contains information about state (USA) and provincial (Canada) licensing for massage therapists. It is current up to the time of publication of this text. Thirty-four of the fifty states license massage therapists at this time. Please check state agencies responsible for licensing or one of the following Web sites for the most current information: www.amtamassage.org; www.abmp.com; www.massagemag.com.

Note: In most states, health care professionals including physical therapists and athletic trainers may perform massage within their scope of practice and in the context of their own license to practice. Check your state for information specific to your situation.

Education required lists only the massage therapy education required. States may also require CPR and other education. Most require graduation from a state-approved or accredited massage school or program. Check state law for the most complete information.

NCETMB refers to the National Certification Examination for Therapeutic Massage and Bodywork (www.ncbtmb.org).

United States
Alabama Massage Therapy Board
610 S. McDonough St.
Montgomery, AL 36104
(334) 269-9990
www.almtbd.state.al.us
Education required: 1000 hours*
Exam: NCETMB

Arizona (Effective date: July 2004)
www.massage.state.az.us
Education required: 500 hours*
Exam: NCETMB

Arkansas State Board of Massage Therapy
103 Airways
Hot Springs, AR 71903
(501) 623-0444
www.state.ar.us
Education required: 500 hours*
Exam: NCETMB or state exam

Connecticut—Massage Therapy Licensure
Department of Public Health
410 Capitol Avenue—MS#12APP
P.O. Box 340308
Hartford, CT 06134
(860) 509-7603
www.dph.state.ct.us
Education required: 500 hours*
Exam: NCETMB

Delaware Board of Massage and Bodywork
Cannon Building
861 Silver Lake Blvd., #203
Dover, DE 19904
(302) 744-4537
www.professionallicensing.state.de.us/boards/massagebodyworks
Education required: 500 hours*
Exam: NCETMB

District of Columbia Massage Therapy Board
Occupational and Professional Licensing Administration
941 N. Capitol St. NE, 7th Floor
Washington, D.C. 20002
(202) 727-7185
www.dcra.org/main.htm
Education from approved school required
Exam: NCETMB

Florida Board of Massage Therapy
Department of Health
2020 Capitol Circle SE, Bin #C09
Tallahassee, FL 32399
(850) 488-0595
www.doh.state.fl.us/mqa/massage/mahome.html
Education required: 500 hours*
Exam: NCETMB

State of Hawaii
Board of Massage Therapy
P.O. Box 3469
Honolulu, HI 96801
(808) 586-3000
www.state.hi.us/dcca/pvl
Education required: 570 hours*
Exam: state exam

Illinois Department of Professional Regulation
320 West Washington St., 3rd Floor
Springfield, IL 62786
(217) 785-0800
www.ildpr.com
Education required: 500 hours*
Exam: to be decided
(Effective date: January 2005)

Iowa Department of Health
Board of Massage Therapy Examiners
Lucas State Office Building, 5th Floor
321 E. 12th St.
Des Moines, IA 50319
(515) 281-6959
www.idph.state.ia.us/licensure
Education required: 500 hours*
Exam: NCETMB

Kentucky Board of Licensure for Massage Therapy
P.O. Box 1360
Frankfort, KY 40601
(502) 564-3296
www.state.ky.us/agencies/finance/occupations
Education required: 500 hours*
Exam: NCETMB

Louisiana Board of Massage Therapy
12022 Plank Road
Baton Rouge, LA 70811
(225) 771-4090
www.lsbmt.org
Education required: 500 hours*
Exam: NCETMB

Maine Board of Massage Therapy
Department of Professional and Financial Regulation
35 State House Station
Augusta, ME 04333
(207) 624-8613
www.state.me.us/pfr/led/massage
Education required: 500 hours*
Exam: NCETMB

Maryland Board of Chiropractic Examiners
Massage Therapy Advisory Committee
4201 Patterson Ave., 5th Floor
Baltimore, MD 21215
(410) 764-4738
www.mdmassage.org
Education required: 500 hours massage* + 60 hours college
Exam: NCETMB

Mississippi State Board of Massage Therapy
P.O. Box 12489
Jackson, MS 39236
(601) 856-6127
www.msbmt.state.ms.us
Education required: 700 hours*
Exam: NCETMB

Missouri Massage Therapy Board
3605 Missouri Blvd.
P.O. Box 1335
Jefferson City, MO 65102
(573) 751-0293
www.ecodev.state.mo.us/pr
Education required: 500 hours*
Exam: NCETMB or approved exam

Nebraska Massage Therapy Board
Health and Human Services
Credentialing Division
301 Centennial Mall South, 3rd Floor
Lincoln, NE 68509
(402) 471-2115
www.hhs.state.ne.us/crl/mhcs/mass/massage.htm
Education required: 1,000 hours*
Exam: NCETMB + practical exam

New Hampshire Office of Program Support
Board of Massage Therapy
Health Facilities Administration
129 Pleasant Street
Concord, NH 03301
(603) 271-5127
www.nhes.state.nh.us/elmi/licertoccs/massa01.htm
Education required: 750 hours*
Exam: NCETMB or state exam

New Jersey Board of Nursing
Massage, Bodywork & Somatic Therapy Examining Committee
P.O. Box 45010
Newark, NJ 07101
www.state.nj.us/lps/ca/nursing
Education required: 500 hours *or* NCETMB
(Effective date: 2003)

New Mexico
Board of Massage Therapy
2550 Cerrillos Rd.
Santa Fe, NM 87505
(505) 476-4870
www.rld.state.nm.us/b&c/massage
Education required: 650 hours*
Exam: NCETMB

New York State Board of Massage Therapy
Cultural Education Center #3041
Albany, NY 12230
(518) 473-1417
www.op.nysed.gov/massage.htm
Education required: 1,000 hours*
Exam: state exam

North Carolina Board of Massage and Bodywork Therapy
P.O. Box 2539
Raleigh, NC 27602
(919) 546-0050
www.bmbt.org
Education required: 500 hours*
Exam: NCETMB

North Dakota Board of Massage
P.O. Box 218
Beach, ND 58621
(701) 872-4895
www.ndboardofmassage.com
Education required: 750 hours*
Exam: NCETMB

Ohio Massage Therapy Board
77 South High Street, 17th Floor
Columbus, OH 43215
(614) 466-3934
www.state.oh.us/med
Education required: 600 hours*
Exam: state exam

Oregon Board of Massage Therapists
748 Hawthorne Ave. NE
Salem, OR 97301
(503) 365-8657
www.oregonmassage.org
Education required: 500 hours*
Exam: NCETMB + practical

Rhode Island Department of Health
Professional Regulation
3 Capitol Hill, Room 104
Providence, RI 02908
(401) 222-2827
www.health.state.ri.us
Education required: 500 hours*
Exam: NCETMB

South Carolina Department of Labor
Licensing and Regulation
P.O. Box 11329
Columbia, SC 29211
(803) 896-4588
www.myscgov.com
Education required: 500 hours*
Exam: NCETMB

Tennessee Massage Licensure Board
Cordell Hull Building, 1st Floor
425 Fifth Ave. N
Nashville, TN 37247
(615) 532-3202
www2.state.tn.us/health/Boards/Massage/index.htm
Education required: 500 hours*
Exam: NCETMB

Texas Department of Health
1100 West 49th St.
Austin, TX 78756
(512) 834-6616
www.tdh.state.tx.us/hcqs/plc/massage.html
Education required: 300 hours*
Exam: written and practical exam

State of Utah Department of Commerce
Board of Massage Therapy
P.O. Box 146741
Salt Lake City, UT 84144
(801) 530-6964
www.commerce.state.ut.us/dopl/wp-app.htm
Education required: 600 hours*
Exam: NCETMB

Virginia Board of Nursing
6606 W. Broadway St., 4th Floor
Richmond, VA 23230
(804) 662-9909
www.vdh.state.va.us
Education required: 500 hours*
Exam: NCETMB

State of Washington Department of Health
101 Israel Rd. SE
Tumwater, WA 98501
(360) 236-4700
www.doh.wa.gov
Education required: 500 hours*
Exam: NCETMB

State of West Virginia
Board of Massage Therapy
200 Davis St., #1
Princeton, WV 24740
(304) 487-1400
www.wvmassage.org
Education required: 500 hours*
Exam: NCETMB

Wisconsin Department of Regulation and Licensing
Massage Therapy Board
1400 E. Washington Ave.
Madison, WI 53703
(608) 266-0145
www.state.wi.us/regulation
Education required: 600 hours*
Exam: state approved exam and NCETMB

Canada
British Columbia
Registered Massage Therapist
(604) 736-3404
Education required: 3,000 hours*

Newfoundland and Labrador
Registered Massage Therapist
(709) 739-7181
Education required: 2,200 hours*

Ontario
Massage Therapist
(416) 489-2626
Education required: two- to three-year program*

active-assisted stretching—A type of stretch in which the athlete moves a joint to its functional limit, followed by the practitioner applying pressure in the direction of the stretch; used to increase strength and coordination.

active palpation—Tactile evaluation of tissue condition while performing massage techniques.

active stretching—A type of stretching performed entirely by the athlete with no assistance.

acute muscle pain—A type of post-exercise muscle soreness thought to be related to ischemia brought by intense exercise of short duration; relieved with massage that increases circulation.

adhesion—A binding together of two anatomical surfaces that are normally separate. Occurs frequently in muscle and connective tissue after trauma or with chronic tension. Deep transverse friction is used to break up adhesions.

beating—A percussion massage technique applied with a lightly closed fist using the hypothenar eminence and small finger as the striking surface; used for stimulation.

body mechanics—The alignment of the practitioner's muscle and skeletal structures to prevent injury when performing massage techniques; good functional posture.

broadening—A massage technique in which muscle and fascial tissue are compressed and widened with a deep, slow, sliding motion; used to break adhesions and increase circulation.

circular friction—A friction massage technique applied in a circular motion covering no more than one square inch at a time; used to mobilize and warm soft tissues and break adhesions.

compression—A massage technique that employs a gradual compressing of tissue followed by a gradual reduction of pressure; used to increase circulation. See *palmar compression* and *digital compression*.

constellation of effects—A theoretical framework for understanding the primary and secondary effects of sports massage. See *primary effects* and *secondary effects*.

contract–relax–stretch—A technique used to enhance stretching by preceding the stretch with a contraction and relaxation of the muscle to be lengthened.

contraindications—Conditions or situations that make receiving massage inadvisable because of the harm that it might do.

cupping—A percussion massage technique applied with "cupped" hands (i.e., fingers pressed together with no palm contact); used for stimulation and loosening respiratory congestion.

debility—A condition that reduces or hinders the athlete's ability to perform a sport, but is not totally disabling. See *remedial applications*.

deep friction—Massage techniques that use short, circular, or back-and-forth motions applied with the fingertip or thumb and using sufficient pressure to produce motion on the tissues beneath the skin; used to treat a specific small area and prevent adhesions.

deep transverse friction—A friction massage technique applied in a direction across the length of the muscle fibers using heavy pressure; used to break adhesions.

delayed-onset soreness—A type of post-exercise muscle soreness that increases from two to three days following strenuous exercise; results in various degrees of stiffness and soreness; relieved with massage that increases circulation.

digital compression—A compression massage technique applied with the thumb or fingertips; used in various kinds of point work (e.g., trigger point, acupressure point, stress point).

disability—A condition that does not allow athletes to perform their sport at all. See *rehabilitation applications*.

doping—The use of prohibited performance-enhancing drugs.

draining—A sliding technique variation in which a limb is placed in a vertical position, and both hands surround the tissue applying deep pressure as they slowly slide from distal to proximal; enhances blood flow in the veins toward the body cavity.

durable hyperemia—Hyperemia that lasts for a long period; one of the goals in pre-event massage. Compression and broadening techniques are often used to induce durable hyperemia. See *hyperemia*.

effleurage—A classic Western massage term for sliding movements; found in Swedish and Russian massage. See *sliding*.

event massage—An application of sports massage in the time period surrounding a competitive event that aims at immediate performance enhancement, recovery, or both. Includes pre-event, interevent, and postevent massage.

faltering effleurage—A combination sliding movement and superficial friction technique in which the hands alternate in short, swift, brushing slides over the skin; has a stimulating effect.

fibrosis—Thickening and scarring of connective tissue due to overuse or injury.

fist placement—Basic hand position for massage in which the dorsal surface of the fingers held in a closed fist are used to apply the massage technique; used for compression and sliding techniques.

friction—Massage techniques in which two surfaces are rubbed over each other repeatedly. See *superficial friction* and *deep friction*.

full-palmar overlay—Basic hand position for massage in which full-palmar placement of one hand is reinforced with the other hand placed on top; used for compression techniques.

full-palmar placement—Basic hand position for massage in which the entire palmar surface of one or both hands applies the massage technique; used for sliding, kneading, and compression techniques.

functional unity—A concept that emphasizes the interconnectedness of the musculature, and that muscles work together in complex ways rather than as separate structures.

general relaxation—A physiological state characterized by decreases in heart rate, oxygen consumption, respiration, and skeletal muscular activity and by increases in skin resistance and alpha brain waves; caused by activation of the parasympathetic nervous system; sometimes called the relaxation response.

hacking—A percussion massage technique applied with the little, third, and fourth fingers, or the side of the hands, with the palms facing each other; used for stimulation.

hyperemia—Increased blood flow to a part of the body. Massage techniques used to induce hyperemia include deep sliding strokes, kneading, and pumping compression.

hyperthermia—A thermal injury that occurs when the core body temperature becomes dangerously high; can result in muscle cramping, heat exhaustion, or heat stroke; signs of hyperthermia include clumsiness, headache, nausea, dizziness, apathy, and impairment of consciousness.

hypertonicity—An increase in muscle tone resulting in muscle tension.

hypothermia—A thermal injury that occurs when the core body temperature becomes dangerously low; early signs of hypothermia include shivering, euphoria, blue lips and nail beds; signs of severe hypothermia include disorientation, hallucination, combativeness, and loss of consciousness.

hypoxia—An insufficient amount of oxygen.

interevent massage—A type of event massage given in the short periods between events in an extended competition that aims at recovery from one performance and preparation for optimal performance in the next event.

ischemia—Insufficient blood flow to tissue that results in decreased oxygen supply (hypoxia), increased carbon dioxide, and an insufficient supply of nutrients. Can cause pain, stiffness, and soreness in the affected area.

ischemic compression—Digital compression, usually with a thumb or single-digit overlay hand position, that causes blanching at the site of application; used for trigger point deactivation, and holding tender points.

jostling—A massage technique in which the soft tissues are shaken back and forth with short, quick, loose movements; may be accompanied by mobilization of surrounding joints; used to loosen up and relax an area.

kneading—A massage movement in which the hands alternately and rhythmically lift, squeeze, and release the soft tissues; used for muscular relaxation and increasing circulation in the tissues; a form of petrissage.

knuckle placement—Basic hand position for massage in which the dorsal surface of the fingers is used to apply massage techniques; open fist; used for compression and sliding techniques.

lymphatic drainage massage—A system of soft, gentle massage techniques used to improve the movement of fluid into the lymph capillaries; used to reduce edema.

maintenance—An all-purpose application of sports massage that is scheduled between competitions. It aims at recovery, normalizing stressed tissues, and treating minor injuries and complaints.

massage—The manipulation of the soft tissues of the body.

massage specialist—A person with special skills in massage and related techniques, gained through education and experience.

massage therapist—A specialist in massage therapy who has graduated from an approved or accredited training program and who, in some states, holds an occupational license as a massage therapist.

multiple-digit overlay—Basic hand position for massage in which multiple-digit placement is reinforced with the fingers of the other hand; used for sliding, friction, and vibration techniques.

multiple-digit placement—Basic hand position for massage in which the tips or pads of several fingers or both thumbs apply the massage technique; used for sliding techniques.

muscle stripping—Deep thumb slides applied in the direction of the muscle fibers, and in parallel strips covering the width of a muscle.

muscle tension—A state of hypertonicity in skeletal muscle usually caused by stress, trauma, or overuse.

muscular relaxation—The opposite of a state of contraction in skeletal muscles. A reduction in muscle hypertonicity induced by massage techniques including sliding strokes, kneading, vibration, and jostling.

NSAIDs—Nonsteroidal anti-inflammatory drugs; for example, acetaminophen (Tylenol), ibuprofen (Advil), naproxen (Anaprox), and aspirin.

optimal therapy zone (OTZ)—The depth at which the massage practitioner must work to have a therapeutic effect; described as the amount of pressure needed to have a therapeutic effect.

palmar compression—A compression massage technique applied with the palm of one hand while hands are in the palmar-overlay position; used to increase circulation to a broad area.

palpation—The skill of identifying anatomical structures and assessing the condition of tissues through touch.

passive-active stretch—A type of stretch in which the practitioner takes a joint to the limit of its functional range, followed by the athlete holding the position for several seconds; used to strengthen a muscle.

passive-resisted stretch—A type of stretch in which resistance is applied by the practitioner prior to a passive stretch; pumping and rocking compression; used along with contract-relax-stretch and reciprocal inhibition techniques.

passive-static stretch—A type of static stretch in which the practitioner applies the technique while the athlete remains passive.

passive stretch—A type of stretch in which the recipient remains passive throughout the movement; performed entirely by the practitioner without the athlete's active participation.

percussion—Massage techniques that employ a rapid, rhythmic hitting movement applied with the hands or fingertips. See *beating, cupping, hacking, pincement, slapping, tapping*. Same as *tapotement*.

petrissage—A classic Western massage term for kneading, lifting, and compression techniques; found in Swedish and Russian massage.

pincement—A percussion massage technique applied with the thumb and fingers in rapid, light, lifting movements on the skin; used for stimulation.

positional release—A noninvasive method used to relax muscles; involves finding tender points and positioning; also called strain–counterstrain.

postevent massage—A type of event massage given after a competition. It aims at enhancing recovery, treating minor injuries and complaints, and responding to health emergencies.

pre-event massage—A type of event massage given from four hours to up to half an hour before competition. It aims at preparing the athlete in mind and body for optimal performance.

primary effects—The direct physiological and psychological effects of sports massage such as improved blood and lymph circulation and reduced anxiety. See *constellation of effects* and *secondary effects*.

prone—Facedown position on a massage table; bolsters are placed under the shoulders and ankles.

proprioceptive neuromuscular facilitation (PNF)—A method of promoting or hastening the response of the neuromuscular mechanism to relax or lengthen a muscle through stimulation of the proprioceptors. See *contract–relax–stretch* and *reciprocal inhibition*.

pumping—Repeated rhythmic palmar compressions that press muscle tissue into the underlying bone; used to create durable hyperemia in pre-event massage.

range of motion (ROM)—The degree of movement of a joint before the movement is impinged upon by surrounding tissues; active or passive movement of a joint through its range of motion for evaluative or therapeutic purposes.

reciprocal inhibition—A physiological phenomenon in which an opposing muscle group (antagonist) relaxes when the agonist group contracts; sometimes used with a stretch of antagonist muscles.

recovery applications—Applications of sports massage after strenuous workouts and competitions to assist athletes in regaining optimal physical and mental condition and reducing the harmful effects of stress.

rehabilitation applications—Applications of sports massage aimed at restoring athletes to normal or near-normal function after a disabling injury; massage as part of a comprehensive treatment plan for a serious injury.

relaxation response—The physiological response associated with activation of the parasympathetic nervous system; includes slower deeper breathing, muscle relaxation, slower heart rate, reduced blood pressure, increased blood flow to internal organs, decreased anxiety, and better sleep.

remedial applications—Applications of sports massage to treat conditions that reduce or hinder athletes' ability to perform a sport, but that are not disabling. See *debility*.

restoration—Restoring an athlete to optimal condition from a state of stress, debility, or disability; includes recovery, remedial, and rehabilitation applications of massage; in Russian literature often means recovery only.

rocking—A joint mobilization technique in which a body part is moved rhythmically from side to side or back and forth; may accompany jostling or compression.

secondary effects—Performance-related outcomes of the primary effects of sports massage, such as fluid movement, greater energy, and faster recovery. See *constellation of effects* and *primary effects*.

session—The application of massage within a specific time period, having a beginning, middle, and end and specific goals; ranges from 15 to 60 minutes. Examples from sports massage include a maintenance session and a postevent session.

side-lying—A position in which the massage recipient is lying on his or her side; the head and upper arm and upper leg are supported with bolsters.

single-digit overlay—Basic hand position for massage in which single-digit placement is reinforced by another finger placed on top; used for digital and ischemic compression techniques.

single-digit placement—Basic hand position for massage in which the tip or pad of a single finger or thumb applies the massage technique.

skin lifting—A massage technique performed by picking up the superficial skin layers and gently pulling them away from underlying muscle tissues.

skin rolling—A massage technique in which the superficial skin layers are lifted from the underlying tissues with a rolling movement from place to place.

slapping—A percussion massage technique applied with the entire palmar surface of the hands or pads of fingers with light slapping movements; often used for stimulation.

sliding—A massage technique that uses a sliding motion (i.e., hands move across the skin with even pressure); used to apply lubricants, for warming and preparing an area for deeper massage, for stretching and broadening muscles, for general relaxation, and as a connecting or concluding technique. See *thumb slide*.

sports massage—The application of massage therapy to athletes and others engaged in intense physical activity for performance enhancement and health maintenance. Sports massage is commonly used for conditioning, recovery, remediation of problem conditions, and rehabilitation; may be scheduled pre-event, interevent, or postevent or between competitions and tournaments.

static stretch—A type of stretch in which a joint is positioned at the limit of its range of motion, and then held for 10-30 seconds; often followed with an increase in range of motion; no bouncing or ballistic movements.

strain—Damage to a part of a muscle, fascia, or tendon brought on by overuse or by overstress; grade 1, 2, and 3 strains vary in severity.

stretching—Joint movement techniques that take joints to their functional limit and then apply pressure in the direction of the stretch; elongates muscle and connective tissue; increases flexibility and range of motion.

superficial friction—A massage technique in which the skin is rubbed briskly for a warming effect; performed with the palms, knuckles, or sides of the hands.

supine—Faceup position on a massage table; bolsters are placed under the knees and neck.

tapotement—A classic Western massage term for percussion techniques; found in Swedish and Russian massage. See *percussion*.

tapping—A percussion massage technique applied with the fingertips or finger pads and typically used in delicate areas such as the face and head; used for stimulation.

tender point—A spot in tense muscle tissue that elicits pain when pressed; used in the positional release technique.

thixotropy—A property of soft tissues by which they become more fluid after movement or when stirred up and more rigid when immobile.

thumb slide—A massage technique applied with the pad of the thumb using a sliding motion to compress muscle and fascial tissue.

treatment—The application of massage for a specific therapeutic purpose.

trigger point therapy—The systematic deactivation of taut tender bands of tissue called trigger points; uses ischemic compression techniques; also called neuro-muscular therapy.

vibration—A massage technique in which the hand or fingertips create a trembling motion; may also be produced by electric vibrators.

wagging—A joint mobilizing technique in which an arm is swung back and forth causing movement in the wrist, elbow, and shoulder of the recipient; performed with the athlete supine and the massage specialist holding the arm above the wrist with the forearm perpendicular to the massage table.

wellness—A dynamic state of health in which a person strives for optimal body–mind well-being.

whole-athlete model—A conceptualization of the athlete as a complex physical, mental, emotional, and social being; theory used to explain the effects of massage for maintaining health and improving sport performance.

Alter, M.J. (1996). *Science of flexibility* (2nd ed.). Champaign, IL: Human Kinetics.

Anshel, M.H. (1991). *Dictionary of the sport and exercise sciences*. Champaign, IL: Human Kinetics.

Arnheim, D.D., & Prentice, W.E. (1993). *Principles of athletic training* (8th ed.). St. Louis: Mosby Yearbook.

Bahr, R., & Maehlum, S. (2004). *Clinical guide to sports injuries*. Champaign, IL: Human Kinetics.

Baumgartner, A.J. (1947). *Massage in athletics*. Minneapolis: Burgess.

Bell, A.J. (1964). Massage and the physiotherapist. *Physiotherapy, 50,* 406-408.

Benjamin, P.J., & Tappan, F.M. (2005). *Tappan's handbook of healing massage techniques* (4th ed.). Upper Saddle River, NJ: Prentice Hall.

Biel, A. (2001). *Trail guide to the body: How to locate muscles, bones, and more* (2nd ed.). Boulder, CO: Books of Discovery.

Birukov, A.A., & Peisahov, N.M. (1979). Changes in the psychological indices using different techniques of sports massage. *Teoriya i Praktika Fizicheskoi Kultury, 8,* 21-24. Translated in M. Yessis, Ed. (1986). *Soviet Sports Review, 21,* 1, 29.

Birukov, A.A., & Pogosyan, M.M. (1983). Special means of restoration of work capacity of wrestlers in periods between bouts. *Teoriya i Praktika Fizicheskoi Kultury, 3,* 49-50. Translated in M. Yessis, Ed. (1983). *Soviet Sports Review, 19,* 4, 191-192.

Boone, T., Cooper, R., & Thompson, W.R. (1991). A physiologic evaluation of sports massage. *Athletic Training, 26,* 51-54.

Bullock, D.M. (1925). *Athletic training methods*. No publisher.

Cash, M. (1996). *Sport & remedial massage therapy*. London: Ebury Press.

Chaitow, L. (1988). *Soft tissue manipulation*. Rochester, VT: Healing Arts Press.

Crosman, L.J., Chateauvert, S.R., & Weisburg, J. (1985). The effects of massage to the hamstring muscle group on range of motion. *Massage Journal,* 59-62.

Cyriax, J.H., & Cyriax, P.J. (1993). *Illustrated manual of orthopedic medicine* (2nd ed.). Boston: Butterworth & Heinemann.

Dixon, M.W. (2001). *Body mechanics and self-care manual*. Upper Saddle River, NJ: Prentice Hall.

Field, T. (2000). *Touch therapy*. London: Churchill Livingston.

Field, T., Fox, N., Pickens, J., Ironsong, G., & Scafidi, F. (1993). *Job stress survey*. Unpublished manuscript, Touch Research Institute, University of Miami School of Medicine. (Reported in *Touch Points: Touch Research Abstracts, 1*[1], 1993.)

Field, T., Morrow, C., Valdeon, C., Larson, S., Kuhn, C., & Schanberg, S. (1992). Massage reduces anxiety in child and adolescent psychiatric patients. *Journal of the American Academy of Child and Adolescent Psychiatry, 31,* 1, 125-131.

Frierwood, H.T. (1953, September-October). The place of health service in the total YMCA program. *Journal of Physical Education, 21.*

Harmer, P.A. (1991). The effect of pre-performance massage on stride frequency in sprinters. *Athletic Training, 26,* 55-59.

Johnson, W. (1866). *The anatriptic art*. No publisher.

Jordan, K.D., & Jessup, D. (1990, Winter). The recuperative effects of sports massage as compared to rest. *Massage Therapy Journal*, 57-67.

Juhan, D. (1987). *Job's body: A handbook for bodywork*. Barrytown, NY: Station Hill Press.

Kaard, B., & Tostinbo, O. (1989). Increase of plasma beta endorphins in a connective tissue massage. *General Pharmacology, 20*, 4, 487-489.

Kelly, D.G. (2002). *A primer on lymphedema*. Upper Saddle River, NJ: Prentice Hall.

King, R.K. (1993). *Performance massage: Muscle care for physically active people*. Champaign, IL: Human Kinetics.

Kresge, C.A. (1983). Massage and sports. In O. Appenzeller & R. Atkinson (Eds.), *Sports medicine: Fitness, training, injuries* (pp. 367-380). Baltimore: Urban & Schwarzenberg.

Lamp, S.P. (1989, Spring). Working in the optimal therapy zone. *Massage Therapy Journal*, 24-25.

Landry, G., & Bernhardt, D. (2003). *Essentials of primary care sports medicine*. Champaign, IL: Human Kinetics.

Manheim, C. (2001). *The myofascial release manual* (3rd ed.). Thorofare, NJ: Slack.

Matveeva, E.A., & Tsirgiladze, I.V. (1985). Use of underwater steam massage and hydroelectric baths in restoration of boxers. Condensed. *Boks, 1*, 28-29.

McKenzie, R.T. (1915). *Exercise in education and medicine* (2nd ed.). Philadelphia: Saunders.

McSwain, G. (1990). *The effect of massage, exercise, and rest on the clearance rate of blood lactate after strenuous exercise*. Unpublished master's thesis, California State University at Fullerton.

Meagher, J. (1990). *Sports massage*. Barrytown, NY: Station Hill Press.

Melzak, R., & Wall, P.D. (1965). Pain mechanisms: A new theory. *Science, 150*, 971-978.

Murphy, M.C. (1914). *Athletic training*. New York: Scribner's.

Namikoshi, T. (1985). *Shiatsu and stretching*. Tokyo: Japan Publications.

Nickle, D.J. (1984). *Acupressure for athletes*. Santa Monica, CA: Health Acu Press.

Persad, R.S. (2001). *Massage therapy & medications*. Toronto: Curties-Overzet Publications.

Pollard, D.W. (1902). *Massage in training*. Unpublished thesis, International Young Men's Christian Association Training School, Springfield, MA.

Rattray, F., & Ludwig, L. (2000). *Clinical massage therapy: Understanding, assessing and treating over 700 conditions*. Toronto: Talus Incorporated.

Rich, G.J. (2002). *Massage therapy: The evidence for practice*. New York: Mosby.

Robbins, G., Powers, D., & Burgess, S. (1994). *A wellness way of life* (2nd ed.). Madison, WI: Brown & Benchmark.

Schultz, R.L., & Feitis, R. (1996). *The endless web: Fascial anatomy and physical reality*. Berkeley, CA: North Atlantic Books.

Sinyakov, A.F., & Belov, E.S. (1982). Restoration of work capacity of gymnasts. *Gymnastika, 1*, 48-51.

Travell, J.G., & Simons, D.G. (1983). *Myofascial pain and dysfunction: The trigger point manual*. Baltimore: Williams & Wilkins.

Travell, J.G., & Simons, D.G. (1992). *Myofascial pain and dysfunction: The trigger point manual, Volume II: The lower extremities*. Baltimore: Williams & Wilkins.

Travell, J.G., & Simons, D.G. (1999). *Myofascial pain and dysfunction: The trigger point manual, Volume I: Upper half of the body* (2nd ed.). Baltimore: Williams & Wilkins.

Werner, R. (2002). *A massage therapist's guide to pathology* (2nd ed.). Philadelphia: Lippincott, Williams & Wilkins.

Williams, R.J. (1943). Second annual national YMCA health service clinic. *Journal of Physical Education, 41*, 30.

Yackzan, L., Adams, C., & Francis, K.T. (1984). The effect of ice massage on delayed muscle soreness. *American Journal of Sports Medicine, 12*, 159.

Yates, J. (2004). *A physician's guide to therapeutic massage* (3rd ed.). Toronto: Curties-Overzet Publications.

Zalessky, M. (1979). Coaching, medico-biological and psychological means of restoration. *Legkaya Atletika, 7,* 20-22.

Zalessky, M. (1980). Restoration for middle, long distance, steeplechase and marathon runners and speed walkers. *Legkaya Atletika, 3,* 10-13.

Web Sites

American Massage Therapy Association: www.amtamassage.org

Associated Bodywork and Massage Professionals: www.abmp.com

United States Anti-Doping Agency: www.usantidoping.org

U.S. Department of Health and Human Services, Centers for Disease Control and Prevention: www.cdc.gov

Note: The italicized *f* and *t* following page numbers refer to figures and tables, respectively.

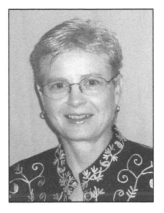

Patricia Benjamin's background as a sport professional for over 30 years gives her special insight into massage for athletes. She has been a high school physical education teacher and coach and a youth sports coach, and she has taught sports at the college level. Her own experiences as an athlete have contributed to her understanding of the benefits of sports massage.

Benjamin received her BS in physical education from the University of Illinois at Chicago and her MS in Education from Northern Illinois University. Her PhD in recreation and leisure studies is from Purdue University, West Lafayette, Indiana.

Benjamin graduated from the Chicago School of Massage Therapy in 1984 and is a licensed massage therapist in the state of Illinois. She is active in the American Massage Therapy Association (AMTA), serving as director of education from 1989 to 1993, and more recently as Illinois chapter president. She is a former AMTA historian and writes a column on the history of massage in the *Massage Therapy Journal*.

Benjamin is coauthor of *Tappan's Handbook of Healing Massage Techniques, Fourth Edition* (2005), teaches professional foundations courses and ethics in massage therapy programs, and is a massage therapy education curriculum consultant and author. She lives in Chicago, Illinois, and enjoys Zen archery, tai chi, history reading, traveling, and gardening.

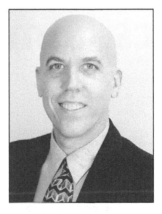

Scott Lamp has been a massage therapist since 1982 and has worked with athletes at all levels. He was the first massage therapist in the United States to be hired by a Division I college athletic association (University of Florida) to provide an ongoing massage therapy program.

Lamp is now the owner and director of Southeastern Sports Massage, a sports massage clinic that develops and implements a variety of projects and programs. He also has his own private practice, which serves more than 30 clients per week ranging from professional athletes to weekend warriors and gardeners. In addition, he develops and teaches certificate programs for sports massage therapy.

Lamp graduated from the Soma School of Massage in Gainesville, Florida, in 1982 and is licensed in the state of Florida. He is nationally certified in therapeutic massage and bodywork. He earned his BS in botany from the University of Florida in 1980.

Lamp has been very active in massage therapy associations, winning numerous awards and serving in many capacities including national president of the American Massage Therapy Association. He has conducted research on the effects of massage as part of a University of Florida research team. Lamp lives in Gainesville, Florida, where his additional interests include house renovation, landscaping, travel, yoga, and watercolor painting.